*B*REAST CANCER

HAS INVADED MY BODY,

BUT IT NEED NOT

INVADE MY SPIRIT.

THERE MAY BE SCARS

ON MY CHEST,

BUT THERE NEED

NOT BE SCARS

ON MY HEART.

—JUDY KNEECE

YOUR

Breast Cancer

TREATMENT HANDBOOK

Your guide to understanding
the disease, treatments,
emotions and recovery
from breast cancer.

Judy C. Kneece, RN, OCN
Breast Health Specialist

EduCare
5150 Ashley Phosphate Rd., Ste. 101
N. Charleston, SC 29418

Fully Revised 6th Edition 2005; 5th Revised Edition 2003; 4th Revised Edition 2001; 3rd Revised Edition 1998; 2nd Revised Edition 1997; 1st Edition 1995
ISBN: 1-886665-22-2
Library of Congress Card Number: 98-093040
Printed in the United States of America
Published by EduCareInc.com

To order:

EduCare
5150 Ashley Phosphate Road, Suite 101
North Charleston, S.C. 29418
800-849-9271 or Fax: 803-796-4150
www.educareinc.com or www.breasthealthcare.com

Illustrations: Debra Strange

Publisher's Cataloging-in-Publication

Kneece, Judy C.
 Your breast cancer treatment handbook: your guide to understanding
  the disease, treatments, emotions and recovery from breast cancer / Judy C. Kneece. — 6th
  ed.
  p. cm. — (EduCareInc.com library series)
  Includes bibliographical references and index.
  LCCN: 98-093040
  ISBN: 1-886665-22-2

 1. Breast—Cancer—Patients. 2. Cancer—Treatment. I. Title. II. Series.

RC280.B8K54 2005   616.99'44906
                            QB101-821

DEDICATION

This book is dedicated to all of the brave women and their families who have faced the pain and emotional recovery from breast cancer and now serve as an inspiration for this handbook.

My appreciation is extended to the hundreds of women and families who shared openly and honestly as I served as their Breast Health Specialist. Their open expression of their fears, questions, challenges and hopes during their breast cancer experience made this book possible. From the privilege of being there with them, I learned the basic education and recovery needs of women diagnosed with breast cancer.

This is also dedicated to the nurses and physicians with whom I have worked and learned. I am especially grateful to Henry Patrick Leis, Jr. M.D., F.A.C.S., dedicated breast surgeon and one of the first pioneers in breast care. He served as my tutor in the medical management of breast disease.

My gratefulness to my support staff that made this updated book a reality: Deanna Lucas, for graphic design and layout; Carrie Phillips, Marilyn Dooley and Nicole Zokan, for editorial services; Debra Strange, medical illustrator; and Melanie Kneece Infinger, Carolyn Brennan and Jody Squallace for their support in all aspects. Their dedication to serve breast cancer patients unselfishly brought this project to fruition.

Someone once asked, "Have you had breast cancer?" My reply was "No, my body has not but my heart has been diagnosed many hundreds of times as I shared the pain my patients were feeling." It is to those of you who now face the same experiences that I make my final dedication. You are the reason for this book!

ACKNOWLEDGMENTS

A special word of appreciation to the following people for their contributions to this work:

Edward P. Dalton, M.D., F.A.C.S., Elliot Hospital Breast Center, Manchester, New Hampshire, Past President National Consortium of Breast Centers

Brian Gelfand, M.D., F.A.C.S., Elliot Hospital Breast Center, Manchester, New Hampshire

Kevin Hughes, M.D., F.A.C.S., Surgical Director, Avon Foundation Comprehensive Breast Evaluation Center, Massachusetts General; Co-Director, Breast and Ovarian Cancer Genetics and Risk Assessment Program; Assistant Professor of Surgery, Harvard Medical School

Cary Kaufman, M.D., F.A.C.S., President National Consortium of Breast Centers, Bellingham Breast Center, Bellingham, Washington

Rosemary Lambert-Falls, M.D., Medical Oncologist, South Carolina Oncology Associates, Columbia, South Carolina

Maurice Nahabedian, M.D., F.A.C.S., Director, Center for Reconstructive Surgery, Johns Hopkins Medical Institutions for review of the reconstruction information.

Ervin Shaw, M.D., Pathologist, Lexington Medical Center, West Columbia, South Carolina, for reviewing the pathology section.

Marianna Maldonado, M.D., Columbia, South Carolina, Psychiatrist and breast cancer survivor, for her insightful expertise in the psychological recovery from breast cancer.

John Coscia, M.D., Radiologist, Executive Director, The Comprehensive Breast Center Don and Sybil Harrington Cancer Center, Amarillo, Texas

Constance Roach, Nurse Practitioner, Avon Foundation Comprehensive Breast Evaluation Center, Massachusetts General

Deirdre Young, RN, OCN, Director of Oncology Services, Lexington Medical Center, West Columbia, South Carolina

Kelly Jeffcoat, RN, OCN, Breast Health Specialist and breast cancer survivor, Lexington Medical Center, West Columbia, South Carolina

Pam DiDente, RN, MN, breast cancer survivor, Community Breast Cancer Case Management for Central Oregon - Sara Fisher Breast Cancer Project, Bend, Oregon

Larry W. Moore, Phar D., SC Oncology Associates, Columbia, South Carolina

Young Survival Coalition for manuscript review.

Harriett Barrineau, breast cancer survivor

Anna Cluxton, breast cancer survivor

Deanna Lucas, Graphic Design and Layout

Debra Strange, Medical Illustrator

TABLE OF CONTENTS

ABOUT THE AUTHOR

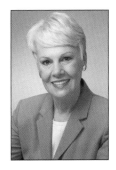

Judy C. Kneece, RN, OCN, is a certified oncology nurse with a specialty in breast cancer and a MammaCare® Specialist. She received training at the Mind/Body Medical Institute of Harvard Medical School. Judy presently serves as an international Breast Health Consultant for hospitals and breast health centers in the educational and psychosocial needs of breast cancer patients and their families. She implements a program of comprehensive education, training nurses to fill the breast health education role and setting up a complete program of support for the entire family unit.

She is also the author of *Helping Your Mate Face Breast Cancer*, a book for support partners and *Finding A Lump In Your Breast—Where To Go . . . What To Do,* which were both reviewed in the Journal of the National Cancer Institute. She has also written *Solving the Mystery of Breast Pain, Solving the Mystery of Breast Discharge* and has created a CD-ROM featuring 353 breast health topics for clinics, hospitals and physicians' offices for individual patient education.

Her background as a Breast Health Specialist working in a hospital served as a catalyst for her insights into the needs of women and their families during the breast cancer experience. Judy has spent much time researching the experience of breast cancer patients by holding national focus groups on the experience of breast cancer, recurrent breast cancer, and most recently on sexuality issues after chemotherapy treatments. Her research serves as a basis for understanding the experience of breast cancer and the needs of patients and their families.

Judy has served as a contributing editor for numerous women's magazines on the issues of breast health and cancer and speaks widely to patients on triumphant survivorship and to medical professionals on the topics of comprehensive breast center strategic planning, patient education and support.

Quoted in *Cope Magazine*, Judy says, "Empowering patients with an understanding of their disease, treatment options and providing tools for recovery management are essential for complete recovery. Breast cancer is more than scars on the breast; it can also scar the heart. We must address the psychological and social issues breast cancer brings if a woman is to successfully manage her disease. An understanding of her disease and personal management skills empowers a woman to become an active partner with her healthcare team and not a passive participant. She must know the advantages and disadvantages of treatment options and the questions she needs to ask about her care. Getting well is more than surgery and treatments; it is a woman understanding the vital role she can play in managing her own recovery."

As survivors, we learn that
survivorship is an attitude we adopt.

It is the one component of recovery
that no one else can do for us.
We have to decide for ourselves
how we intend to respond
to our illness and how
we approach our recovery.
We, alone, decide to
become survivors.

— *Judy Kneece*

Each individual decides whether
and how he or she will grow from
an experience of suffering.
Perhaps your decision already has been
clearly made. Perhaps you've said to
yourself, "I am determined that
I"m going to learn from my loss."
If you have made such a decision,
your healing is not just underway—
it's a foregone conclusion!

—*Anne Kaiser Stearns*

DEAR SURVIVOR:

I almost began this letter "Dear Patient," but then I changed my mind. I do not want you to see yourself or think of yourself as only a patient. You will be a patient for only a short time. You will be a survivor for the rest of your life. I want you to know that you are, from the innermost parts of your being, a breast cancer survivor.

Painful as the diagnosis must be, you have joined a host of other women who have experienced the overwhelming anxiety of hearing the words "You have breast cancer" and are now living examples of survivorship. Among those survivors are:

- Olivia Newton-John
- Jill Eikenberry
- Betty Ford
- Ann Jillian
- Justice Sandra Day O'Connor
- Betty Rollin
- Peggy Flemming
- Carly Simon
- Julia Child
- Linda Ellerbee
- Kate Jackson
- Shirley Temple Black
- Happy Rockefeller
- Diahann Carroll
- Nancy Reagan
- Evelyn Lauder
- Marcia Wallace
- Cokie Roberts

As you can see from this list, although breast cancer is an unwelcome experience, it is one that can add depth and influence to your life. These well-known women are now advocates in education and support for other women living with cancer. As you begin your journey to understand and recover from breast cancer, be assured that you, too, can master the experience. You can learn, as they learned, how to take the crisis of breast cancer and transform it into an opportunity for personal growth. You can become a triumphant survivor.

As an oncology nurse working only with breast cancer survivors, I have had the privilege to share the intimate experiences of the breast cancer journey with hundreds of women. They shared many of their needs, fears and questions about their disease, treatment and recovery. They also shared many tips which made the experience much easier for them. In this book, I have attempted to share with you the best of what I learned from the patients and physicians with whom I worked.

There is much to know about your disease and recovery. This book is designed to serve as a basic primer for this information. It is not meant to replace or supplant your physicians' instructions. Your physicians and nurses will add additional information and suggest reading materials to help you. Surviving cancer starts with understanding what you can do now that you have cancer. By learning about your disease, you are beginning your journey to survivorship like millions of other women.

Best wishes for a happy and healthy future,

Judy

THE VOICES OF EXPERIENCE:

As I worked with newly diagnosed breast cancer patients, I quickly learned the value of their early interaction with other women who had experienced breast cancer. They needed to talk to a peer who had survived all of the decisions that they were going to have to make over the next weeks and months. While writing this guide for you, I immediately decided to include other women's experiences with breast cancer so that you too could benefit from what they have learned. To serve as your peers throughout this book, two women from very different situations share their experiences, fears and thoughts on their journeys with breast cancer. Let me introduce you to Harriett Barrineau and Anna Cluxton.

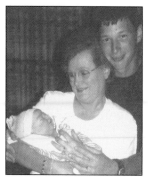

Harriett, her son Chris and grandson Blake

"To me, this picture is what survival means."

HARRIETT'S STORY

Harriett was diagnosed with breast cancer in 1991 at the age of 44. At the time of diagnosis, she was married and had four sons. Today she has four daughter-in-laws and eight grandchildren. Harriett says, "This is what survival means."

Because of the characteristics of her tumor, she had a modified radical mastectomy, and followed her surgery with chemotherapy. Over a year later, the resulting posture shift caused back pain and spurred Harriet's decision to have a prophylactic second mastectomy and immediate bilateral reconstruction.

As a Breast Health Educator, I had the opportunity to work with Harriett. She often shared her fears, feelings, failures and triumphs during her breast cancer experience. Her honest and insightful reflections during her diagnosis, treatment and recovery are a source of comfort to other women who are just beginning their journeys. Harriett openly shares with other women what she has experienced. She tells them that they will not always feel hopeful and that there are going to be problems, but that with determination, they too can make it. She is the epitome of survivorship—the quality of using present coping skills and learning new skills to triumph over a seemingly insurmountable task.

Today, Harriett works full-time in her husband's accounting firm and has served as a Reach to Recovery volunteer. Harriett remembers how after her diagnosis, she searched for people who would share with her the ins and outs of the experience.

Harriett's quotes in this book serve as the voice of one who personally knows the perils of the journey you are undertaking; she is a woman who has been where you are and where you are going—a woman who has survived! Al, her husband, provides the same type of commentary in the book *Helping Your Mate Face Breast Cancer*, written for support partners.

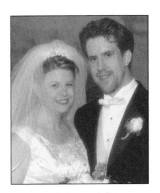

Anna and Brian on their wedding day

"Too young for breast cancer . . . but I learned from experience that breast cancer does happen to young women."

ANNA'S STORY

Anna was 32 years old and single when she noticed a flattened area below her left nipple. She performed monthly breast self-exams, but she had never felt anything different in this area. Gradually, she noticed that the area would flatten out more when she raised her arm. Anna mentally dismissed it as hormonal changes or recent weight loss, but continued to keep her eye on it. She had other important things to do—she was planning her wedding.

The wedding went as planned without any problems. She and her new husband, Brian, went to Jamaica for their honeymoon. During the trip, she noticed that she could now feel a lump under the flattened area of her breast. When they arrived home, she called her OB/GYN, who performed an ultrasound. The doctor immediately decided a mammogram was needed. Anna saw a surgeon and had a fine needle biopsy seven days after she had been sitting on the beach in Jamaica. Twenty minutes after the biopsy, she was told that it looked positive for cancer. "Brian and I were completely shocked," Anna told me. "I can't even remember what else the doctor said to us after those words."

One month after the wedding, Anna underwent seven hours of surgery for a mastectomy with an immediate TRAM flap reconstruction. All 16 lymph nodes removed during the surgery came back negative. Anna had chemotherapy. The day of her first chemo treatment, Brian shaved his head to show his support. "When other couples are supposed to be starting their new life together, Brian was sitting on the bathroom floor holding me as I was throwing up."

Anna recalls the experience: "Cancer changed our lives as individuals and as a couple. I was young—too young for breast cancer, some would think. But I learned from experience that breast cancer does happen to young women. I also learned that having cancer at an early age brings different types of problems to a woman and her spouse. Because of this, I am now active in the Young Survival Coalition, which educates and supports young people with breast cancer, addressing the problems that cancer brings. I also work for breast health services at the same hospital where I received my treatment. I interact daily with other women hearing the same words I heard—the biopsy is positive for cancer."

Anna and Brian's life changed quickly. They were a very young couple facing a breast cancer diagnosis, but they allowed an unexpected visitor to turn their lives into a mission to help others. I asked Anna to share how a young woman thinks and responds to the different decisions that have to be made. Throughout this book, you will read Anna's response to her cancer diagnosis as a young woman. Brian provides the same type of commentary in the mate's book, *Helping Your Mate Face Breast Cancer*.

SURVIVORSHIP

Loss has a way of changing our
lives dramatically.
We become transformed.
However, the idea that learning
and personal growth could come from
our loss when we are in the middle of our
pain is an almost disgusting idea.
This is how most people feel
the first six months or longer.
It takes time and we have to
move past our crisis to see
the changes that have occurred.

—*Anne Kaiser Stearns*

As survivors, we take a
misfortune of life and change
it into something that produces personal
growth and somehow benefits others.

As survivors, we choose hope after loss.
We choose to look at what we can do now
that cancer has invaded our lives.
We acknowledge our loss and nurse our
pain, but we move on to make the
diagnosis a source of motivation for a
new direction in our lives.

— *Judy Kneece*

THE EMOTIONAL IMPACT OF BREAST CANCER

"My emotions were on a constant roller coaster ride. One minute I was so grateful I had a good prognosis. Then anger, fear and depression took over. I realized I was going to need help working through my emotions."

—HARRIETT BARRINEAU
SURVIVOR

Understanding Your Emotions

Shocked. Scared. Angry. Disappointed. Numb. Irate. Crushed. Disarmed. Brokenhearted. Furious. Speechless. Overwhelmed. A complete loss of control over my life. These are all terms women have used to describe their emotions upon hearing the words, "You have breast cancer." Most women report that little was heard or remembered after the words "you have breast cancer" were spoken. Their fears took control as they recalled all that they knew in the past about breast cancer. Most thought, "Will I die?" Often, they remembered someone who had gone through a similar diagnosis, and mentally they substituted themselves into the role. In the midst of this mind-boggling experience, the physician informed them of surgery options and possible treatments. "Overwhelmed" is usually an inadequate word for the experience. How do you begin to work through this complicated maze of emotions and unexpected decisions you have to make?

Foremost, you must realize that breast cancer is usually a very treatable disease. Survival rates are at an all-time high. Strong emotions are normal for all women at this time. Fears are natural. Most importantly, you need to know that breast cancer is usually not a medical emergency. You can take several weeks without endangering your health to sort through your emotions and seek answers to your questions. Your physician will discuss the appropriate time frame with you. Use this time to gain an understanding of the treatment options you have and the advantages and disadvantages of each. It will be best for you, both emotionally and physically, to take the time to make informed, rational decisions about your treatments.

"I didn't process everything for a few days after hearing I had breast cancer. Then several days later, at six o'clock in the morning, I had an emotional meltdown. Having my husband there to comfort me helped. But I also needed time by myself to reflect on what was happening to me. I had an unplanned future to consider."

—ANNA CLUXTON
SURVIVOR

What is a Normal Response?

Women experience an array of emotions and respond to the diagnosis according to their basic personalities and previous life experiences. Common to all is that this is a new experience, one that demands a great deal of physical and emotional energy. Most women cry and face depression as they sort through their potential losses. Remember, tears are okay. They confirm that you are dealing with reality and are using a very natural and appropriate response to deal with loss. Do not deny yourself the right to grieve. Grieving and tears are signs that your emotional healing has begun.

Some women experience great anger. This anger may be directed against themselves for not taking steps toward an earlier diagnosis, or toward a physician or even a family member. Anger is an emotion that is used to try to regain control over a situation in which control has been lost. Usually, it serves as a non-productive way to solve problems; however, it is a natural response. A sense of control will return as you begin to understand and learn about the disease and how you can participate in your recovery. Loss has to be acknowledged before steps to recovery can be effective.

Communicating with Family and Friends

Eventually, your thoughts will turn from yourself to your family and friends and the effect your diagnosis will have on them. They, too, are in emotional pain over your loss. The diagnosis is also a shock to them. Like you, they have a need to express their sad feelings, usually by crying, feeling down and questioning what is ahead as they grieve with you over your loss. This is also a necessary and natural part of the family's emotional adjustment to your diagnosis.

You can play a vital part in facilitating their recovery by talking openly of your feelings and allowing them to ask questions and express their thoughts. This is probably one of the hardest parts of the breast cancer experience—open, honest communication. If honest communication begins at the time of diagnosis, it will help both you and your family. Often, we think that if we say nothing or do not let anyone see us crying or feeling depressed, we are making it easier for other people. The opposite is true. Being dishonest and not talking about feelings creates an atmosphere of uncertainty. People don't know what to say or do, and this results in increased anxiety among family members.

Positive attitudes are needed. However, attitudes that seem overly optimistic may block communication in families because they set the stage for everyone to be in denial and mask their feelings. The family also needs to see you express your full range of emotions and be able to do so themselves. Begin to share as soon as you can, and ask them to share with you. They may need your permission before they talk because they don't want to "upset" you. They want to help you through this time. When you talk openly, they can find ways and actions that will best help you. Help them to be a part of your recovery by allowing them to do things for you. For example, when they offer to do a chore, accompany you to the doctor or do something special for you, accept the offer. Feeling useful helps facilitate their emotional healing.

Communicating during times of stress may not be easy. You may find it difficult to open up and talk. The one closest to you may not respond if you open up and share. Breast cancer doesn't change your basic personality or emotional responses to life. If you, your mate or other family members, found it difficult to talk before the diagnosis, it may still be difficult to share during this time. However, you need someone with whom you can openly share your thoughts and fears in an understanding, nonjudgmental atmosphere. Since you can't force people to participate in communicating, it may be necessary for you to look outside the family unit for someone who can best respond to your needs. Consider your friends, a professional counselor or a support group. It is necessary and helpful for you to locate a support system in which you will be free to communicate and share your feelings, whatever they may be. You need a safe place to talk where your feelings, thoughts and fears will not be criticized or condemned but will be listened to instead.

Studies have shown that women who have good support systems adjust and respond to treatment more effectively. Ask your physician or clinic nurses for names of counselors or support groups for breast cancer patients in your area. Breast cancer support groups provide a safe and helpful environment where you can share, learn and receive support from women who know exactly how you feel and what you are facing. The American Cancer Society or Komen Foundation will also have a list of groups that meet in your area. Find somewhere to communicate your feelings! Acknowledging your emotional responses as normal and communicating openly will set the stage for a successful emotional recovery.

Getting the Facts Straight

Often family and friends who are trying to be helpful will offer you information and suggestions concerning your surgery and treatments. They do this because they care. However, this may only serve to confuse you and increase your anxiety. It is best to listen but not let this interrupt your quest to learn specific information concerning your diagnosis from the professionals guiding your treatment. There have been great advancements in the treatment and management of breast cancer. Drugs have been designed that have changed many of the side effects of chemotherapy. Surgical treatment is often less disfiguring because of newer surgical procedures, and survival rates are at an all-time high.

Learning about your disease, surgeries and treatment is important in order to regain a sense of control in your physical recovery. Breast cancer is a disease with many variables. There are approximately 15 types of breast cancer, many that require different surgical management and treatment. For this reason, you cannot compare notes with a friend who had breast cancer or listen to well-meaning family or friends because there are too many differences in treatment. Your information needs to come from someone who knows your exact diagnosis and has up-to-date information on the medical management of your disease. Your physician and healthcare staff will be the best source for accurate information.

Managing the Breast Cancer Experience

As you are communicating and actively learning about your disease, you will find yourself experiencing mood swings. There will be periods when you feel that you are doing well. Then you may find that you once again feel overwhelmed, asking "Why?" and "What did I do to deserve this?" or saying, "I don't think I can go through this." These are normal responses as you are working through a crisis. You won't always feel in control. Feelings of depression, with periods of crying, may be dispersed throughout your recovery. When these times occur, don't be too hard on yourself for not being "brave." Acknowledge them as normal and then take steps to restore your positive mood by doing whatever seems to help. For some, it helps to get out of the house for a special outing, spending time with friends or working on a hobby. You should take steps, whatever helps, to regain a positive mood.

It is also necessary that you monitor your rest during this time. A crisis can drain us of normal energy and require that we get more rest. Listen to your body and get adequate rest. Most women need seven to eight hours of uninterrupted sleep daily. This may mean that you have to ask family members to assume some of your household duties for a time. Plan to include fun events. It is important to do things you enjoy. This will reduce stress as well.

Breast cancer is not an event you would have invited into your life. You will need to learn how to best participate with your healthcare team in your recovery, but don't allow yourself to make a "career" out of cancer. Try to see it as an experience to rekindle your life. Many women believe that the breast cancer experience caused them to grow into happier and healthier women, adding new dimensions to their lives that they had never taken time to enjoy before. Look at this time as an opportunity to grow, learn and make positive changes in your life. Consider an exercise program. Change your nutritional habits, or take time to start a hobby that brings you joy. A crisis can serve as an opportunity to grow into a physically and emotionally stronger and happier individual. Seek to make this a time of personal growth.

No matter how bewildering and uniquely
painful we privately think our situation is,
somehow there is solace in knowing that
the experiences felt after a diagnosis
are universal and common to most women.

Emotional recovery from cancer is a
process. It is better to think of it
as a recovery journey.
Some days just putting one foot in
front of the other is progress.
Sometimes you may feel that others have
gone through the process more quickly
while you find yourself struggling.
But remember, recovery is an individual
journey and you cannot compare
yourself with others.
This is your recovery journey.

Asking for help or support after a cancer
diagnosis is often very hard for us to do.
We find it much easier to be the one to give.
Receiving is hard. Asking for help is even
harder. However, allowing others to help
us gives them a sense of self-worth
through being of help to us.

— Judy Kneece

RELATIONSHIP WITH YOUR MATE

"I needed reassurance from my husband. I needed to hear, 'I love you.' I needed attention from him. His faith had to be strong enough for both of us for a short time. But, later, I realized he also needed support. He, too, was hurting. He found this unique source of understanding in a mates' support group."

—HARRIETT BARRINEAU
SURVIVOR

At diagnosis, your mate is confronted with the same surprise and faces the same overwhelming emotions as you. Yet, in the midst of all of this, they often strive to be strong, understanding and supportive. The way your partner responds to this crisis will also be determined by their basic personality and previous coping experiences. Behaviors may vary among people, but under it all are the basic emotions of fear, loss and uncertainty. A mate's love for you causes a strong emotional experience and an extreme feeling of helplessness when you are diagnosed with breast cancer. This is one thing they cannot fix. In an interview concerning support partners, Dr. Marilyn T. Oberst stated:

*Learning to live with cancer is no easy task. Learning to live with someone else's cancer may be **even more difficult**, precisely because **no one** recognizes just how hard it is to **deal** with someone else's cancer.*

Communicating With Your Mate

It is difficult to see you, the one they love, suffering emotionally and physically. Some mates may withdraw their emotions quietly as they mentally sort out the situation. They may not say anything. Others may be very verbal. Remember, this is a new experience for them also. They too are hurting emotionally and often feel inadequate in their responses. You can help them by sharing your needs **verbally**. Do not wait, hoping that they will know what you need them to do or **how** you wish for them to

"I was so afraid of what having 'damaged goods' for a wife would do to our young marriage. It became very important to both of us to know when to reach out to each other and when to let go."

—ANNA CLUXTON
SURVIVOR

respond. Most mates want to meet their partners' needs and be helpful, but they are not sure how to respond. Recent studies by Dr. Oberst show that during the first six months, some mates may experience greater degrees of emotional problems after a diagnosis than the patient because of personal fears and the anxiety created by not knowing what is expected of them in their new role as a support partner. You can help by encouraging your mate to talk to others who understand the role of a support partner. Call your cancer treatment center or local American Cancer Society office for the name of support groups for partners or ask for the name of a volunteer. Chaplains working in cancer treatment centers are an excellent source of support because of their understanding of the unique stressors that families face with a cancer diagnosis. Encourage your mate to reach out to others to meet their own personal needs.

Changes in the Intimate Relationship

"What effect will my diagnosis and surgery have on my intimate relationship?" "Will I still be loved?" "How will my new body image affect our sexual relationship?" These thoughts are in the back of most women's minds. They are valid questions that need to be explored and understood. Intimate relationships are built on mutual love, trust, attraction, shared interests and common experiences in life. Breast cancer will not change these shared feelings.

What may change is how you view your body and how that can affect your sexual intimacy. The physical aspect of lovemaking may temporarily change because of loss of energy resulting from your treatments. However, you can resume your sexual relationship as soon as you feel able. You are still the same person your mate selected and loves. You can bring a new dimension to this relationship by openly discussing your feelings about the changes in your body image. Try to communicate honestly about these concerns.

Often, you will need to be the one to initiate the discussion of these fears or needs. Your mate may feel these issues are too personal or sensitive. It is helpful if these concerns are addressed as soon as you are diagnosed. Allowing time to pass only makes the conversations more difficult and walls of silence easier to build.

Early viewing of your incision area is very helpful in restoring the relationship and preventing distance between you and your partner. After surgery, you may feel embarrassed or afraid to talk about your changed body image or to be seen nude by your mate. These feelings are best confronted and faced early. Viewing the incision is a necessary step. It has been proven that, if you share openly, these feelings can be overcome. Accepting the changes and reaffirming your love and joy of being alive and together will help you work through these feelings.

Mates often fear that their physical closeness may cause pain or injury to the incision site. It is helpful for you to share your need for physical closeness and what is comfortable or uncomfortable to you. Many times what women mistakenly sense as sexual rejection is really an effort on the part of the mate to protect the one they love. Therefore, state your desire for physical contact and share what is pleasurable. This will reduce the unspoken fear in your mate's mind concerning physical intimacy.

Open communication will decrease anxiety for both you and your mate, enabling your personal and sexual relationship to grow even stronger. There may be a period of adjustment, but most couples put their fears behind them and reestablish a satisfying and loving relationship. By sharing both the troubles and triumphs of cancer openly, you and your partner will have the opportunity to strengthen bonds of affection, trust and commitment.

Changes in the Family

Cancer is a family affair. It emotionally affects every member of the family. A cancer diagnosis is similar to throwing a stone into a body of water. The stone causes ripples that are greatest to those closest to the person diagnosed and diminishing in intensity to those further away emotionally. Naturally the mate and the children feel the greatest impact. However, extended family and friends are also impacted. An essential part of healing and recovery is allowing each person to handle the pressures in a way that matches their basic coping skills. Some will be very talkative and want to come and share this time with you. Others may find themselves without words and withdraw emotionally for fear of not knowing what to say. It is helpful if you remember, that like you, this is a new experience and they have to process their response over time. Cancer presents not only a challenge to family unity, but also an opportunity to strengthen bonds and increase love, respect and understanding. Studies report that most family relationships improve or become closer after a diagnosis.

Support Partner's Guide Available

A companion to this book, *Helping Your Mate Face Breast Cancer*, is available for your support partner. This book is designed as a guide to help a mate understand how to best help you while understanding their own emotional responses to the diagnosis. It addresses the unique emotional issues that a mate faces during a partner's breast cancer diagnosis and explains what they can do. Ask your healthcare provider about this book, or you may order it from EduCareInc.com or at the address provided in the back of this book.

REMEMBER

Your mate suffers emotionally from the diagnosis, just as you do.

Most mates are unsure about how best to help. Helping them adapt to the role of support partner requires open communication. You must let your mate know how to best help during the experience by verbalizing your needs and expressing your desires.

Encourage your mate to reach out for support from others who understand the unique needs of a support partner.

Intimate relationships are based on love, trust, shared interests and common experiences; breast cancer does not change this.

Sexual intimacy after surgery is dependent upon open communication. Discuss your change in body image, view the incision early and verbalize your need for continued intimacy.

Breast cancer can bring a couple closer and strengthen the bonds of affection, trust and commitment.

The entire family is affected by your diagnosis. All members will respond differently according to their personalities and previous coping skills.

Grief over losing something that

is important cannot be legislated.

It is important that we allow our

feelings of grief to exist.

It is normal, even necessary,

to express our feelings to trusted people.

For a time it is helpful to admit

our bewilderment, our anger, our

uncertainty and our fears of the future.

This helps our emotional healing.

If we force ourselves to deny these

feelings we are only compounding

our problems.

Find a trusted person and talk about

your disappointments you are facing.

Openness can be a good first step toward

resolving the seemingly impossible

task of moving forward.

— *Judy Kneece*

TELLING YOUR CHILDREN

"Having always been the caretaker in my family, I found it difficult to let my four sons know I needed anything. I finally told them that I needed to talk about my fears and feelings, even though talking about Mom's breasts was not the most comfortable subject. Our love for one another and deep faith in God brought us closer together during this crisis."

—HARRIETT BARRINEAU
SURVIVOR

Children react to a parent's illness in various ways, according to their ages, developmental stages and personalities. As a parent, you want this illness to create as little negative effect as possible on their lives. How do you handle this situation so that it causes the least amount of emotional distress for your children? From the beginning, tell the truth and answer their questions honestly. Often, it may appear that keeping the facts from them would be more helpful, but this is not wise. Children are very perceptive; they instinctively sense when something is wrong in the family. Not knowing what is wrong will often cause them to imagine things, which results in more anxiety than knowing the truth. It is also important that they hear it first from you or the family, not from strangers. When information is presented truthfully, on their level of understanding, they can interact with you and receive answers to their questions and fears. It may be helpful to ask your medical team if they have information on how to talk with children about cancer.

Tips for Telling the Children:

- If possible, wait until you and your mate have some control of your emotions. For some, this may take a day or two; others may be able to share the first day.

- Ask your treatment team for information, or call your local American Cancer Society for information written for children about a parent's cancer.

- With your mate or family member, plan what you will say to the children. Plan a time when both of you can share with them and not be interrupted.

- Turn off the television and hold telephone calls to prevent interruptions.

- Start by sharing something similar to the following: "Mommie has found a lump in her breast. The doctor says that the lump is cancer (call it by the right name). Cancer cells grow too fast. The doctors say that they need to take this lump out because these are not good cells. The doctors and nurses can also help by giving medicine." Continue to share truthfully and simply what the facts are. If you have an example that will help explain, this will be helpful.

- If you or your mate begins to cry, assure your children that this is because you are sad and it is okay to be sad and to cry.

- Allow the children to ask questions. Answer to the best of your ability. If you do not know the answers, be honest and say you do not know.

- Reassure them that you will continue to tell them what is happening.

- Involve them in the process of helping Mom adjust to surgery and possible treatments. Help them to feel as if they are part of the solution to the problem by sharing chores that contribute to the well-being of the family.

Teenage children and grown children also need to communicate openly and honestly. However, don't be surprised if they don't seem to be overly concerned and quickly return to their normal duties and interests. Take this as a compliment; your openness has restored their confidence that, as a family, you can cope with your new situation.

It is suggested that you inform the teachers or instructors of your children that your child is dealing with a cancer diagnosis (or family crisis) at home. This alerts them and allows them to identify potential changes in a child's behavior as a stress reaction to the change in their home environments. This knowledge allows them to offer support and understanding if a child should act out, rather than correction. They will also be able to recognize if the child is suffering from overwhelming sadness and needs emotional support. Older children and teens may feel more comfortable sharing their feelings with adults outside the home rather than with their parents. This information allows this person to offer valuable emotional support to your child.

Teachers are also often in a position to request help and assistance from other school personnel, such as trained professional counselors and school psychologists, in order to offer additional professional emotional support to a child.

Impact of Diagnosis on Children

In his book, *How Do We Tell The Children?*, David Pertz, M.D., explains:

> *A child's first question about illness and death is an attempt to gain mastery over their frightening images of abandonment, separation, loneliness, pain and bodily damage. If we err on the side of overprotecting them from emotional pain and grief with 'kind lies' we risk weakening their coping capacities.*

In her article, *Children of Parents with Cancer*, found in the *Journal of Psychosocial Oncology: 1992*, Karen Greening MSW, LCSW, summarizes a child's five basic needs during a parent's diagnosis:

- A need for a clear information on what is happening

- A need to be involved and to help out

- A need for realistic reassurance

- An opportunity to express their thoughts and feelings

- A need to maintain their normal interests and activities

Families often worry about the effect the illness will have on their children. The most important factor in how they respond is how they see you and your partner respond to the illness. If they see you communicating openly, honestly, and sharing with a positive attitude, they will be more likely to respond the same way. The family can value this time as one of growth and maturity in problem solving. If you find it difficult to know what to say or realize problems are developing in the family with the children, contact your cancer treatment center and ask for a counselor trained in dealing with children.

REMEMBER

Children need to be told the truth, at
the level of their understanding, by
you or a close family member.

They need their questions
answered honestly.

Truthfulness, coupled with love,
will enable your child to grow
stronger through this family crisis.

Children need to feel a part
of the family by assisting with
household chores.

Teens need to maintain their
social life as much as
possible and not become
the only source of
communication or support
for the parent.

Breast cancer does not have
to be a negative experience
for children. It can serve as a time
when families grow stronger.

SURVIVORSHIP

You gain strength, courage and
confidence by every experience in which
you really stop to look your fear in the face.
You are able to say to yourself,
"I have lived through this horror.
I can take the next thing that comes along."
You must do the thing you
think you cannot do.

—*Eleanor Roosevelt*

Many of our fears are tissue paper-thin,
and a single courageous step would
carry us right through them.

—*Brendan Francis*

Courage is not the lack of fear.
It is acting in spite of it.

—*Mark Twain*

CHAPTER 4

CALMING YOUR FEARS

"My husband's first reaction to my diagnosis was that we had been given a death sentence. Mine was just the opposite. I saw death as the easy choice. My greatest fear was having to live with the aftermath of breast cancer."

—HARRIETT BARRINEAU
SURVIVOR

Fear is a paralyzing force. As a nurse working with breast cancer patients, I have listened to the many fears that a diagnosis brings. Often the fears become overwhelming as they are realized. In our support group, women are often surprised to hear other women express the same fears. Yes, most fears women have are common to all. However, they may vary in degrees of intensity according to your personality, previous coping experiences and your present support system. The most commonly expressed fears are:

- Will I die?

- How do I need to plan for the future?

- Are they telling me the truth?

- Will I live to see my children grow up?

- How can I protect my loved ones from the pain this causes?

- Can I cope after I have my breast removed?

- Will treatment be painful?

- Will treatment work?

- How will I know if cancer recurs?

- I feel helpless. What can I do about cancer?

"I remember coming across a Web site about a young woman who died from breast cancer and it scared me to death. Until that moment I don't think I had made the actual connection in my mind that I could die from this. Talking to my doctors and getting honest answers helped me put everything into perspective."

—ANNA CLUXTON
SURVIVOR

How do you handle your fears? First, know that fear is natural. In fact, women who do not express fear are those who are most at risk psychologically. Disarming fear begins with recognizing its presence, expressing the fear to the appropriate person and taking steps of action against the fear. Do not hold on to your fears in silence. Identify your fears and express them. Often, when fears are expressed, strategies can be developed to help you to deal with your fear.

Make a list of the fears that are clouding your mind (see the example below). Be honest. You do not have to show anyone the list. After you have made your list, in a column beside the fear, list the people or person that the fear involves. If another person is involved, such as your mate or physician, express your fear to them. Think about the fear and actions that you can take to understand or to change it.

FEARS	PERSON(S) INVOLVED	THINGS I CAN DO
"Will I still be sexually attractive?"	Mate	Express fear Purchase attractive lingerie Express desire for closeness Plan for special times
"Are they telling me the truth?"	Physician/ Nurses	Ask for honesty and all the facts Read about my disease
"What can I do about living with cancer?"	Support Group Professional Counselor	Attend a support group Ask for the name of a counselor

A worksheet for listing your fears and your planned strategies to disarm them is located on page 199. Begin by listing your fears. When you are ready to express your fears to the appropriate person, state your fear questions using "I" language. Example: "I am very concerned about the effect of my surgery on our sexual relationship. I don't want it to change." You may say to your physician, "I want to know all of the details about my disease and the side effects of treatment."

Fear can be a great impediment to recovery. Expressing the fear, determining your resources and developing a plan of action will cause the fear to be less of a threat. Communicate openly with your healthcare team and your support partners. Verbalizing the fears allows them to help you seek a strategy to deal with the fear. Not all uncertainty will be alleviated, but the fears can certainly be brought to a manageable level.

Sources that have proven to assist in the management of fear are support groups, professional counselors and spiritual faith. From these sources a wealth of strength may be gained to deal with the diagnosis of cancer. As your physician and healthcare team are working to eradicate the cancer from your body, you can work to provide an emotional environment in your body as free from stress and fear as possible.

Support Groups

Support groups are a "safe" place to express your fears and have your cancer questions answered by those who truly understand. You may have loving support from your family and friends, but often they do not seem quite able to understand what you really feel. In a breast cancer support group, the shared experiences of other women serve to restore the adaptive process needed to resume your fighting spirit. It is helpful to see those who are months ahead of you living full, productive lives after mastering the crisis of breast cancer. They have many tips and much encouragement to share with you. Avail yourself of this source of strength and understanding.

Ask your treatment team for names of groups or call your local American Cancer Society or Komen Foundation. When you have identified a support group or groups, you may wish to call and ask about the organization and goals of the group. Select a group that is affiliated with a medical facility, if possible. These groups are usually facilitated by professionals who have an understanding of breast cancer and are able to get accurate answers to your questions.

Visit the group at least twice before making a judgment. If you do not feel you had your needs met, visit another group if possible. Try to avoid any group that is allowed to become a "pity party" and select one which offers education and sharing among participants and promotes an optimistic approach to recovery.

It is also helpful if your mate can attend a support group. Often, mates have very few people with whom they can confide and receive helpful support. Ask about local support groups for your mate. A companion to this book for support partners, *Helping Your Mate Face Breast Cancer*, is available as a support guide from EduCareInc.com, offering tips on how mates can aid in their role as supporters.

Some cancer centers also offer educational classes for younger children. This allows them to meet with other children and learn about cancer and cancer treatment on their level of understanding. Ask about children's classes for educational support.

Most patients feel that support groups were helpful to their recovery. Women who participate in groups or seek support from professionals have been proven to adjust more quickly both physically and emotionally than non-participants. Support groups are a way to reduce your fears and get answers to your questions.

Professional Counseling

Support groups are a valuable source of free information and support. However, some women do not feel comfortable in a large group or do not have access to a support group because of time or distance. If you find that a support group cannot meet your needs, ask your healthcare team for the name of a specialized counselor, therapist or psychiatrist. This is not a sign of weakness but of strength. Seeking appropriate support is as necessary as seeking appropriate medical treatment. The difference is that you may have to express your need for this service.

Individual counseling allows you to express your feelings and fears in an atmosphere of trust and support. Your selected counselor helps you plan strategies to make this crisis a manageable event in your life. This is usually short-term crisis counseling.

Spiritual Faith

Inherent in each of us is a deep need for understanding our existence and our future. Cancer causes a real threat to our sense of safety and forces these issues to be foremost in the mind. Answers to your struggles to understand "why," "how" and "what about tomorrow" are found in one's faith. It will be helpful if you reach out and seek the help of your spiritual counselor during this time. If you do not have a pastor, priest, rabbi or spiritual leader, ask your hospital for the name and number of their chaplaincy service. Chaplains are trained in dealing with the adjustment to the crisis of cancer. Avail yourself of this valuable service.

In the book *Cancervive*, Susan Nessim shares her feelings as a cancer survivor:

Cancer has taken us on an amazing journey. When we look in the mirror we may see our faces as unchanged, but the person they belong to has undergone a spiritual metamorphosis. We have shed our old skins. Now we must assess who we've become and where we're headed. . . . We've gained new insights into the depths of our spiritual strength, physical resiliency and courage.

Looking at the cancer experience through the eyes of spiritual faith gives the experience meaning and purpose. Susan continues,

In the school of life, cancer survivors feel as if they've just completed an accelerated course—not that anyone, given the choice, would sign up for that course again. But for those fortunate enough to have gained a new perspective, the lessons learned are as precious as life itself.

Why Do I Keep Losing It Emotionally?

Feelings and fears are a lot like holding on to Jell-O. Just when we think we have them in our hands and under our control, they ooze out or slip right out of our grasp.

This is the natural course of dealing with a crisis. We are not always in control of our feelings. We may think we are doing well and handling our emotions. Then, seemingly without warning, new problems arise, fears of the future return, tears begin to flow and depression comes to visit. Dealing with a cancer diagnosis is not an easy task. It keeps bringing new problems and fears as you progress through treatment and recovery. If you feel that your emotions slip out from under your control at times, you are normal. Most people dealing with a cancer diagnosis have this happen. When it does, you just have to start all over and look behind the cause of your present fears and see what, if anything, you can do. Don't be too hard on yourself. You don't have to be a superwoman.

Refer to Tearout Worksheet
Managing My Fears - Page 199

REMEMBER

Fear is common to all women diagnosed with breast cancer.
You are not unusual because of your fears.
Relax—you are normal.

Fear is not a sign of weakness.

Keep in mind that fears vary in intensity according to
an individual's personality, previous coping
experiences, and support systems.

Fears lose their power when expressed openly
and when steps are taken to disarm them.

The first step is to name the fears and
questions that cloud your mind. Write them down.

Support groups offer much emotional help
and answer many fears and questions.

Some women are not comfortable in a large group
and can benefit greatly from individual
professional counseling.

Spiritual faith is a strong component in giving meaning to fear
and providing a sense of strength to surmount the crisis of
diagnosis. Reach out for spiritual understanding.

Keeping control of our emotions is often like holding on to
Jell-O. Sometimes they ooze out or slip from our
control for a while. This is normal.

"Fighting fear is like trying to sack fog; you just can't get a
handle on it. Giving your power away to the fear is worse
than suffering the consequence that you're afraid of.
Choose to give yourself the chance.
It's normal to be anxious and afraid,
but you can't be dominated by the fear."
Dr. Phil McGraw, *Life Strategies*

SURVIVORSHIP

I have a lot of things to prove to myself.
One is that I can live life fearlessly.

—*Oprah Winfrey*

Fear is conquered by action.
When we challenge our fears,
we defeat them.
When we grapple with our difficulties,
they lose their hold upon us.
When we dare to face the
things which scare us, we
open the door to freedom.

—*Wynn Adams*

As survivors, we remember that
even horrible losses can be
transformed into learning.
We decide, even in the midst
of our pain, to learn from our loss.
We move from the question
of "Why me?" to
"Now that this has happened,
what shall I do about it?"

—*Judy Kneece*

WHAT IS
BREAST CANCER?

"Breast cancer is not the unconquerable enemy I thought it was."

— HARRIETT BARRINEAU
SURVIVOR

"'Know thy enemy'—what an understatement. I learned so much about cancer in the first few weeks after my diagnosis. And I continue to learn as much as possible, as this is an unending battle!"

—ANNA CLUXTON
SURVIVOR

Breast cancer is not a sudden occurrence, but a process that has been developing for a period of time. Therefore, when a biopsy confirms a cancerous breast tumor, you are most often not facing a medical emergency. You have time to get answers to your questions and learn about your particular disease and treatment options. Most physicians recommend surgery within several weeks of biopsy. There are exceptions; for example, inflammatory carcinoma requires immediate treatment with chemotherapy for maximum control. Ask your physician what recommendations will be made regarding your particular tumor. Tests performed on your tumor will reveal cell type and estimate whether the tumor is a very slow growing or a more rapidly growing tumor.

Some tumors will characteristically spread more rapidly to other parts of the body, while others do not spread as quickly. Breast cancer spreads to other parts of the body through the lymphatic system or the blood system. The spread of cancer can be local (in the area of the breast), regional (in the nodes or area near the breast) or distant (to other organs of the body).

What Causes Breast Cancer?

The female breast is a very complicated glandular organ and is the site of the most common cancer in women—breast cancer. No one knows exactly what causes breast cancer. Genetics, having a family history of breast cancer, increase the risk. Other identified possible causes have been environmental carcinogens, viruses, and radiation. Promoting factors identified are lifestyle factors, including diet and hormonal function.

Cancer begins when the cells of the breast undergo changes. The normal cell is damaged and converts into a cell that has an uncontrolled growth pattern. The cancer cells continue to divide and grow and may spread to other parts of the breast and then to other parts of the body if not removed. The cancer cells can invade neighboring tissues and spread throughout the body, establishing new growths at distant sites. This process is called metastasis.

INTERNAL STRUCTURE OF THE FEMALE BREAST

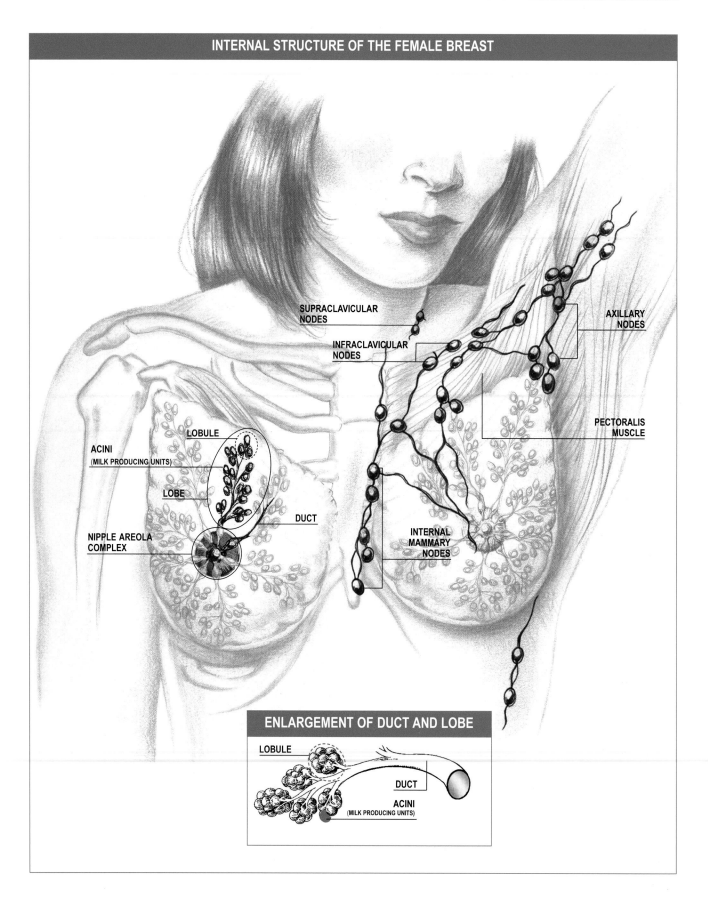

SUPRACLAVICULAR
NODES

INFRACLAVICULAR
NODES

AXILLARY
NODES

PECTORALIS
MUSCLE

LOBULE

ACINI
(MILK PRODUCING UNITS)

LOBE

DUCT

NIPPLE AREOLA
COMPLEX

INTERNAL
MAMMARY
NODES

ENLARGEMENT OF DUCT AND LOBE

LOBULE

DUCT

ACINI
(MILK PRODUCING UNITS)

Types of Breast Cancer

Cancers are first classified according to their relationship to walls of their origin. The two major divisions are **in situ** and **invasive/infiltrating**.

NORMAL LAYER OF CELLS	IN SITU CANCER CELLS	INVASIVE CANCER CELLS

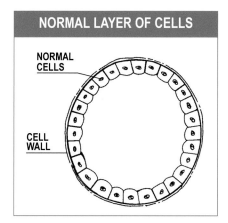

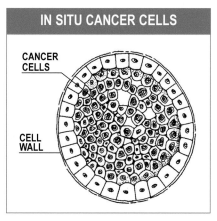

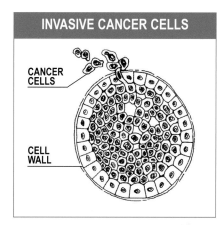

Normal ducts and lobules are lined with one or more layers of orderly cells.

In situ carcinomas are cancers that are still contained within the walls of the portion of the breast in which they developed. The cancer has not grown through the cell wall and invaded surrounding tissue.

Infiltrating or **invasive** carcinomas are cancers that have grown through the duct or lobular walls and into surrounding tissues.

Approximately 15 different types of breast cancer have been identified. The term carcinoma is used by physicians to describe a malignant or cancerous growth. Tumors that develop from different types of breast tissue, in different parts of the breast, may have varying characteristics of development.

Breast cancers are named according to the part of the breast in which they develop. Cancers beginning in the ducts are called ductal carcinomas and comprise the largest number of cancers occurring in women. Cancers beginning in the lobules are called lobular carcinomas and account for a small percentage of diagnoses. In situ carcinomas are cancers that are still contained within the walls of the breast area in which they developed. They have not invaded surrounding tissue. If the cancer grows through the cell walls it is called an infiltrating or invasive carcinoma.

DESCRIPTIONS OF CANCER

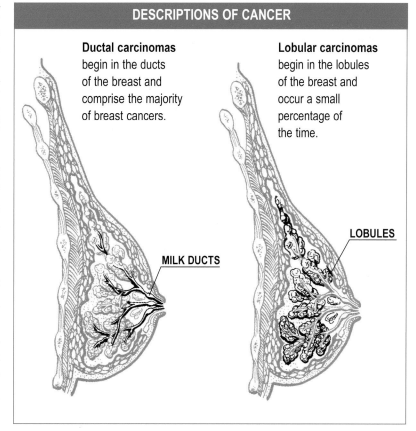

Ductal carcinomas begin in the ducts of the breast and comprise the majority of breast cancers.

Lobular carcinomas begin in the lobules of the breast and occur a small percentage of the time.

MILK DUCTS

LOBULES

INVASIVE AND IN SITU CANCERS

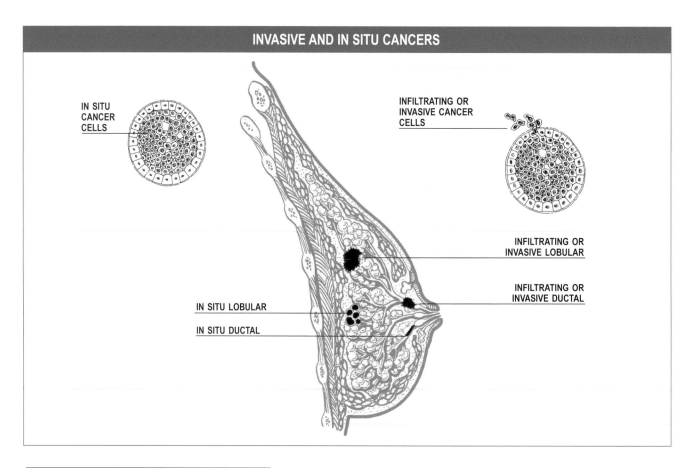

IN SITU CANCER CELLS

INFILTRATING OR INVASIVE CANCER CELLS

INFILTRATING OR INVASIVE LOBULAR

INFILTRATING OR INVASIVE DUCTAL

IN SITU LOBULAR

IN SITU DUCTAL

FREQUENCY OF OCCURRENCE

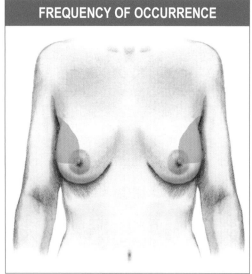

Most breast cancers occur in the upper, outer part of the breast, near or in the area from the nipple back toward the underarm area (axillary tail). Interestingly enough, more cancers occur in the left breast than in the right breast.

Cancer Growth Rate

Some cancers grow rapidly, while others grow very slowly. Breast cancers have been shown to double in size every 23 to 209 days. A tumor which doubles every 100 days (the estimated average doubling time) would have been in your body approximately eight to ten years when it reaches about one centimeter in size (3/8 inch)—the size of the tip of your smallest finger. The cancer begins with one damaged cell and doubles until it is detected on mammography or by finding a lump or other symptom. The cancer must be surgically removed from the body, killed with chemotherapy or radiation therapy or controlled with hormonal therapy. Some people believe that cancers may grow in spurts and the doubling time may vary at different times. However by the time a one centimeter tumor is found, the tumor has already grown from one cell to approximately 100 billion cells.

DOUBLING RATE OF CANCER CELLS

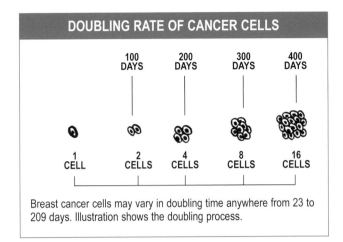

| | 100 DAYS | 200 DAYS | 300 DAYS | 400 DAYS |

1 CELL · 2 CELLS · 4 CELLS · 8 CELLS · 16 CELLS

Breast cancer cells may vary in doubling time anywhere from 23 to 209 days. Illustration shows the doubling process.

TUMOR GROWTH RATE

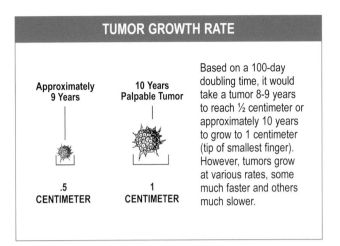

Approximately 9 Years — .5 CENTIMETER

10 Years Palpable Tumor — 1 CENTIMETER

Based on a 100-day doubling time, it would take a tumor 8-9 years to reach ½ centimeter or approximately 10 years to grow to 1 centimeter (tip of smallest finger). However, tumors grow at various rates, some much faster and others much slower.

The Role of the Lymphatic System

Lymph nodes play an important role in the discussion of your treatment decisions. It is helpful if you understand how the lymphatic system affects many decisions. The lymphatic system serves as the sewage system for cellular waste in the body. The lymph vessels follow closely beside the blood vessels and receive the cells' waste products. This waste is carried by the vessels and filtered through rounded areas of the lymph system, referred to as lymph nodes. Nodes appear as small, round capsules and vary from pinhead to olive size. Lymphocytes and monocytes (cellular components of fluid which fight infection) are produced in the nodes, and the nodes act as filters to stop bacteria, cellular waste and cancer cells from entering the blood stream. Lymph nodes may serve as metastatic sites—places where cancer has spread from the original site to nodes, now referred to as secondary sites.

The majority of the lymphatic fluid leaving the breast is drained through the nodes located in the area of the armpit, referred to as the axillary nodes. A small amount is drained through the lymph nodes located in other areas of the breast and the breast bone, called internal mammary nodes. For identification purposes, nodes are divided into three levels in the breast. Your surgeon may remove nodes from one or several levels.

A procedure called axillary sampling is a process in which nodes are taken from under your arm. Axillary dissection is a procedure in which all the nodes under the arm are removed, usually from levels one and two. The number of nodes in each level varies from person to

person. Nodes are removed to determine whether your cancer has moved from the breast into the node area. The term negative nodes means that your lymph nodes did not have any evidence of cancer. Positive nodes indicate that the cancer was found in the lymph nodes. Your surgeon will tell you how many nodes were removed during your surgery and how many were found to have cancer cells present. Treatment decisions are often based

LYMPH NODES OF THE BREAST

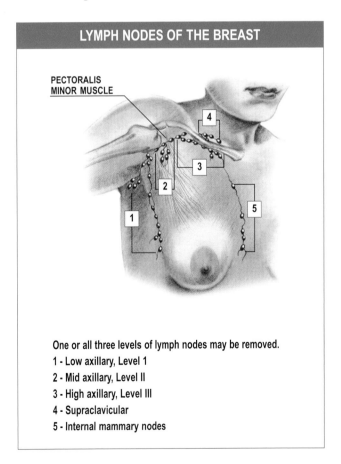

PECTORALIS MINOR MUSCLE

One or all three levels of lymph nodes may be removed.
1 - Low axillary, Level 1
2 - Mid axillary, Level II
3 - High axillary, Level III
4 - Supraclavicular
5 - Internal mammary nodes

on the number of nodes in which cancer cells are found. Two important factors that determine your oncologist's treatment plan are the number of positive nodes and the size of your tumor.

Sentinel Lymph Node Mapping and Surgery

Sentinel lymph node mapping is a procedure that identifies the first nodes (sentinel) that receive lymphatic fluid from a cancerous tumor, thus identifying the lymphatic drainage pattern. The sentinel nodes are like the gatekeepers to the rest of the lymph nodes. Lymphatic fluid contains white blood cells, proteins, and fats that pick up the cellular waste of tissues and then flow through the nodes, which act as filters. Because this fluid passes through these nodes, the lymphatic system is a major route by which cancer spreads or metastasizes. Cancer cells can reach the lymphatic system and filter through the nodes where they multiply. They may pass also through the lymphatic system into the bloodstream. (See lymph node illustration on previous page)

Tumors may drain to different node chains, according to the position of the tumor in the breast. The procedure identifies the lymphatic chain and the nodes most likely to indicate whether cancer has metastasized to the regional lymph node area. This identification gives the surgeon and pathologist a reliable guide for more accurate node evaluation without removing a large number of nodes. Sentinel node surgery may not be available in all surgical centers. Ask if it is available in your center.

This procedure begins with an injection of a radiographic substance before going to surgery. Before surgery begins, the surgeon injects a blue dye around the tumor site or areola; it is carried by the lymph fluid to the closest node(s) (sentinel). During surgery, a hand-held gamma-detection probe first identifies where the radiographic material has concentrated, showing the area for the surgeon to make the incision. The blue dye helps the surgeon visually identify the node (there may be one or several) for removal. After surgery, the pathologist examines these nodes for cancerous cells. (Some surgeons may only use the dye.)

Sentinel node mapping improves the accuracy of selecting nodes to be removed surgically for evaluation to check for the spread of the cancer. It may also prevent unnecessary removal of nodes not in the lymphatic drainage field of the tumor. Reducing the number of nodes removed can greatly decrease the potential for future lymphedema (a swelling from lymphatic fluid accumulation in the arm, which can cause discomfort and is a lifetime risk) and the likelihood of an infection in the arm if any type of injury should occur.

Pregnant women, women with known positive nodes, certain size tumors, women with ductal carcinoma in situ (DCIS), or women with more than one tumor in the breast may be ineligible. Your surgeon will inform you if you are a candidate.

Summary

Surgery and treatment with chemotherapy, radiation therapy or hormonal therapy can all vary because of the differences in types of cancer, the size of the tumor, potential lymph node involvement or documented metastasis, aggressiveness of the tumor and hormonal sensitivity. Therefore, it is necessary for you to communicate with healthcare professionals who have access to your final pathology report when seeking any specific information or advice on your breast cancer treatment.

Refer to Tearout Worksheets
Personal Healthcare Provider Records - Page 209
Personal Treatment Record - Page 211

REMEMBER

No one knows exactly
what causes breast cancer.

Breast cancer is not a sudden
occurrence; it has been
developing for years.

Breast cancer is usually
not a medical emergency.
Most often you have time to gather
information and get answers to
your questions before surgery
or treatments begin.

Don't compare your breast cancer
diagnosis with the diagnosis of others.
There are approximately
15 different types of breast cancer.
Treatment options will vary.

There are many treatment decisions.
The right decision is the one you
feel most comfortable making.

Information gathering is necessary
and good to do after a cancer diagnosis.
However, we can become paralyzed
in gathering information.
It is the action we take that
makes the difference.

The storms of life cause the oak trees
to develop deeper roots.
Life's problems cause us to become
stronger and more sensitive human
beings if we take the opportunity to
grow and learn from our experiences.

—*Judy Kneece*

There is little difference in people . . .
the little difference is attitude.
The big difference is whether it
is positive or negative.

—*Clement Stone*

SURGICAL TREATMENT DECISIONS

"I was frightened by how fast things were happening. I felt totally ignorant about breast cancer and had no idea where to turn for information or education."

—HARRIETT BARRINEAU
SURVIVOR

"I had a limited amount of time to make my surgical decisions. I made my decisions after talking with my healthcare team and based my decision on what I felt was the best choice for me. I couldn't look back or have regrets."

—ANNA CLUXTON
SURVIVOR

When your acute emotional stress is diminished, you may have many concerns about your diagnosis that need to be clarified. Many women say they were not prepared to hear the diagnosis and that everything the doctor said after the word "cancer" was hazy in their minds. You may want to list your questions and call the physician's office to schedule an appointment to receive accurate answers to your questions. Make this list with the person who accompanied you to the initial appointment. Before your visit, it will be helpful to begin reading and acquiring a basic understanding of the medical terms used and some of the treatment options that may be offered. This book contains this basic information. Your physician or nurse can recommend other books or brochures that will be helpful.

Today, women have the opportunity to participate and decide, with their physicians, which type of treatment will meet their personal needs and give the best chance for disease-free survival. It is important for you to understand why you are, or are not, offered certain treatment modalities. As an informed patient, you can become an active partner with your physician, understanding the treatments being discussed. It is also helpful if you can select one support person to accompany you to your appointments and participate in this process. This person will be a shoulder you can lean on and can help you remember and evaluate the information that is presented.

Obtaining accurate information about your particular disease is very important. Ask your physician for recommended reading material. Women's magazines contain much information that is interesting, but it may not apply to the type of cancer you have and may confuse you. Medical terms sometimes have unusual meanings. Using a glossary to clarify the definitions of words will be helpful. As you read and learn, a sense of understanding will replace much of your fear about breast cancer. (Listed at the end of this book are sources of free medical information that offer up-to-date material on breast cancer. Also listed are suggested reading materials and resource lists to assist you in other areas, in addition to a glossary of breast cancer terms.)

Treatments for breast cancer are local (breast only) treatments and systemic (pertaining to the entire body) treatments. Local treatments include surgery and radiation therapy. Systemic treatments are chemotherapy and hormonal therapy; these treatments travel to all parts of the body. Each type of treatment will be discussed in following chapters.

During your evaluation for breast cancer treatment you may have a variety of physicians involved in evaluation of your cancer. Each has a special expertise in treating breast cancer. Refer to tearout worksheets located in the back of the book for a list of questions to ask each physician.

- **Radiologist**—physician who uses diagnostic techniques such as mammography, ultrasound and minimally invasive biopsy to diagnose cancer.

- **Pathologist**—physician who analyzes cells or the characteristics of the tumor removed from your body to determine if disease is present.

- **Surgeon**—physician who removes identified area of suspicion from the body by using surgery.

- **Reconstructive (Plastic) Surgeon**—physician who reconstructs altered or removed breast using body tissues or implants.

- **Medical Oncologist**—physician who specializes in internal medicine and in the treatment of cancer using a variety of methods including chemotherapy, immunotherapy and hormonal therapy. Your surgeon may have an oncologist evaluate you for cancer treatment before or after your surgery. It is very important that you have a good relationship with your oncologist if you are to receive other treatments in addition to your surgery. There will be a need for a great deal of interaction between you and the oncologist during the time you are receiving treatments. You should feel comfortable asking questions and participating in treatment decisions with your oncologist. Refer to Chapter 10 for a complete discussion on the role of the oncologist, chemotherapy and hormonal therapy.

- **Radiation Oncologist**—physician who specializes in using radiation (x-ray) therapy to treat local areas of disease. If your physician feels that radiation therapy could kill any remaining cancer cells in an area of your body, you will be referred to a radiation oncologist. Most breast conserving surgeries are followed by radiation therapy. If you are having radiation therapy, it is helpful to have a consultation with the radiation oncologist before your surgery. Refer to Chapter 11 for a full discussion of radiation therapy and the questions you may wish to ask during your consultation.

Determining Factors for Surgery

Surgery is the first line of defense against most breast cancers. Your surgeon will discuss with you the best surgical options for your diagnosis. Your surgeon will consider the following facts in determining which surgery best suits your needs:

- **Type of tumor**—The type was diagnosed by biopsy and confirmed by the pathology report. There are approximately 15 cell types of breast cancer that vary in tumor growth rate (how aggressively the tumor may spread to other organs and its potential for occurring in the other breast).

- **Size of the tumor**—Sizes are given in centimeters (cm) and millimeters (mm). (10 mm equal 1 cm; 1 cm equals 3/8 inch; 1 inch equals 2.5 cm)

- **Size of your breast**—Some breasts may be too small in comparison to the size of the lump to give good cosmetic appearance when the lump is removed.

- **Location in your breast**—Tumors under the nipple sometimes will not give a suitable cosmetic look when the lump is removed. Two tumors in the same breast not located close to each other will not give good cosmetic results.

- **Lymph Nodes**—Possible tumor involvement in lymph nodes.

- **Mammogram**—Determines if your tumor may be multifocal (occurring within one quadrant in the breast) or multicentric (occurring in more than one quadrant in the breast). This is sometimes evidenced by microcalcifications (small calcium deposits) or mammographic abnormalities.

- **Involvement of other structures**—skin, muscle, chest wall, bone or other organs.

- **Reconstruction**—Your desire for reconstruction now or later and the desired outcome for the reconstructive surgery (breast enlargement, reduction or matching present size).

- **Health**—Your general health and any treatment limitations due to your present health.

- **Disease Control**—Which surgery will give you the best chance for disease control.

- **Cosmetic Results**—Which surgery will give you the best cosmetic results.

- **Range of Motion**—Which surgery will give you the best functional results for your arm and shoulder.

- **Complications**—Which surgery is associated with the fewest short-term and long-term complications.

- **Personal Desire**—Your priorities regarding the surgery.

Treatment for each tumor must be evaluated in terms of its unique and specific features and what surgery will be best for you. Some types of breast cancer may require chemotherapy treatments before surgery, called neo-adjuvant chemotherapy. Discuss the above considerations with your surgeon and ask any questions that will help you make the decision best suited to your needs.

Types of Surgery

Surgery for breast cancer includes several types of surgical procedures. Some types remove the breast (mastectomy), and others remove the tumor and varying degrees of the remaining breast tissue (lumpectomy). These common terms may describe various amounts of tissue removal, and you will need to clarify with your surgeon which of the exact procedures will be used. Following, are the basic types of surgical procedures and descriptions of the

tissues usually removed. After each description, one drawing illustrates the amount of tissue removed, and another drawing illustrates how your body will appear after the surgery. Surgical incisions can vary with different surgeons. A graphic is provided at the back of this book (page 204) for your surgeon to draw the procedure that will be used for your surgical treatment and how your scar should appear afterwards.

Breast Conservation Surgery (Lumpectomy)

Surgery that conserves your breast is commonly referred to as a "lumpectomy." Breast conservation surgery preserves your body image because it saves the majority of the breast tissue, including the nipple and the areola. However, there are some reasons that breast conserving surgery may not be the best surgical option.

Factors That May Disqualify You for Breast Conserving Surgery:

- Pregnancy (if radiation therapy will be required before delivery; surgery is possible in the third trimester if radiation can be given after delivery and starting within six weeks of surgery)

- More than one primary tumor in the breast

- Mammogram with evidence of suspicious scattered microcalcifications

- Location of the tumor in the breast where there may be poor cosmetic results (example: when the tumor is located under the nipple, unless reconstruction is used)

- Size of tumor (if the tumor is too large or the breast is too small in relation to the size of the tumor, then there will be poor cosmetic results)

- Prior radiation therapy to breast or chest area

- Collagen vascular disease (lupus, scleroderma, etc.)

- Severe chronic lung disease (because you may not be a candidate for radiation therapy)

- Very large pendulous breast (may indicate you may not be a good candidate for radiation therapy; you need to have a radiation oncologist's evaluation)

- Evidence of remaining cancer in ducts surrounding tumor after surgical removal (indicating there may be a high risk for recurrence)

- Inability of surgeon to obtain clear margins (no evidence of cancer) after re-excision of area

- Identified carrier of a BRCA1 or BRCA2 mutated gene

- Restrictions on travel or transportation to clinic for daily radiation for five to seven weeks

Lumpectomy Procedures

There are several types of breast conserving surgeries. Different amounts of tissue may be removed according to the size and cell type of your tumor. These variations in the amount of tissue removed have different names. Lymph node removal during breast conserving surgery also varies. Ask your surgeon which of the procedures will be performed and the extent of tissue and lymph node removal you will need to have. There is a separate page (page 204) that your surgeon may fill in for you as to where and how your incision will look after your surgery. The different breast conserving surgeries are defined below:

1. Lumpectomy

Lumpectomy removes the tumor and a small wedge of surrounding tissue. Lymph nodes may or may not be removed by a separate incision under your arm.

Incisions for breast conserving procedures appear very similar in relation to the cosmetic appearance of the breast, differing only in accordance to the amount of tissue removed.

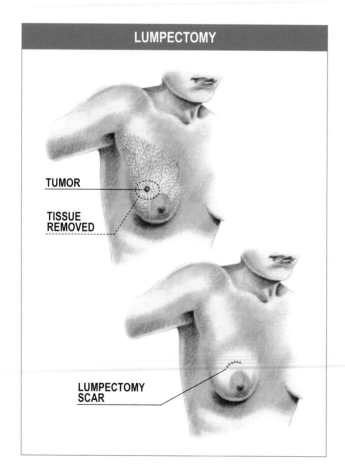

LUMPECTOMY

TUMOR

TISSUE REMOVED

LUMPECTOMY SCAR

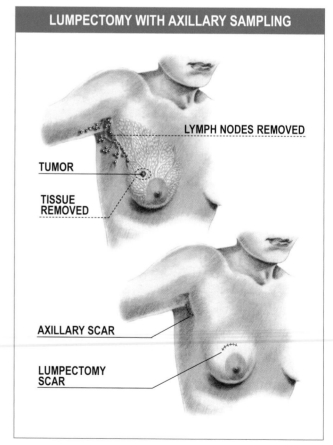

LUMPECTOMY WITH AXILLARY SAMPLING

LYMPH NODES REMOVED

TUMOR

TISSUE REMOVED

AXILLARY SCAR

LUMPECTOMY SCAR

2. Tylectomy

The tumor and a wide area of tissue around the tumor are removed during surgery. Lymph nodes may or may not be removed by a second incision under the arm.

3. Partial or Segmental Mastectomy

The tumor, possibly the overlying skin, and an area of tissue around the tumor are removed in this surgery. A portion of the lining of the chest muscle under the tumor may also be removed. Lymph nodes may or may not be removed from a separate incision, approximately two inches in length, under the arm.

Ask your physician what type of lymph node evaluation procedure is recommended for your breast conserving surgery.

Mastectomy Procedures

There are several types of mastectomies. Ask your surgeon which of the procedures will be performed and the extent of tissue and lymph node removal you will need to have. There is a separate page (page 204) in the back of this workbook that your surgeon may fill in for you, outlining where and how your incision will look after surgery. The different mastectomies are defined below:

1. Full or Complete Radical Mastectomy

A complete radical mastectomy removes the breast, nipple, areola, all three levels of lymph nodes, small chest muscle, the pectoralis minor, medial pectoral nerve and the lining over the chest wall muscles.

TYLECTOMY / PARTIAL SEGMENTAL MASTECTOMY

TYLECTOMY

TUMOR

TISSUE REMOVED

PARTIAL MASTECTOMY

TUMOR

TISSUE REMOVED

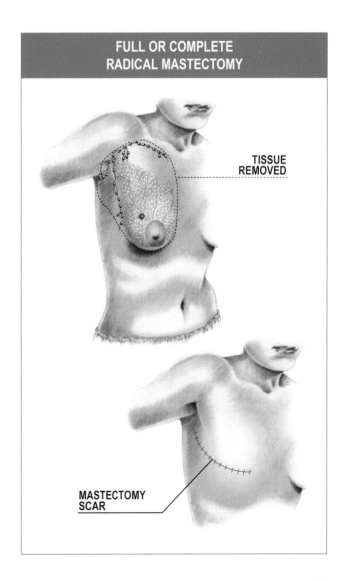

FULL OR COMPLETE RADICAL MASTECTOMY

TISSUE REMOVED

MASTECTOMY SCAR

2. Modified Radical Mastectomy

A modified radical mastectomy removes the breast, nipple, areola, underarm lymph nodes and the lining over the chest wall muscles. You may hear the procedure referred to as a "total mastectomy with axillary dissection," which means that the entire breast and some or all of the level one and two lymph nodes are removed. The chest muscles and pectoral nerves are not removed.

3. Total, Simple or Prophylactic Mastectomy

This procedure removes the breast tissue, nipple, areola, and possibly some of the underarm lymph nodes that are closest to the breast.

TOTAL, SIMPLE OR PROPHYLACTIC MASTECTOMY

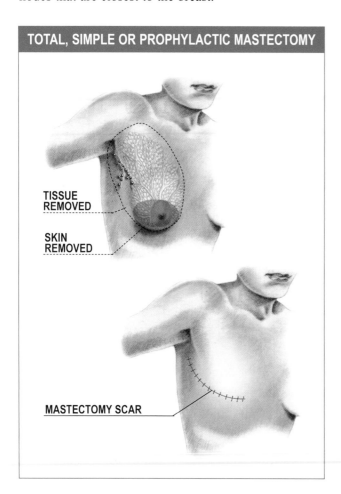

TISSUE REMOVED

SKIN REMOVED

MASTECTOMY SCAR

4. Skin-Sparing Mastectomy

Skin-sparing mastectomy is a procedure used when performing a simple or total mastectomy. The method removes the breast tissues from a circular incision around the areola (dark colored circle). The nipple, areola, breast tissues, nodes located near the breast tissues and additional lymph nodes are removed according to the discretion of the surgeon. The procedure is often selected when reconstructive surgery is performed. The sparing of the skin allows reconstructive surgery to be performed with little need for a period of stretching of the skin. Sensitivity of the skin over the reconstructed breast remains intact. The reconstructive incision is made using the normal curve of the breast. This incision is not visible because it is hidden under the fold of the breast and is concealed by the bra. The incision used to remove the breast is concealed by the reconstruction of a nipple and areola. This is the recommended surgery for women having mastectomy for intraductal disease and desiring reconstruction or for a small peripheral tumor.

SKIN-SPARING MASTECTOMY

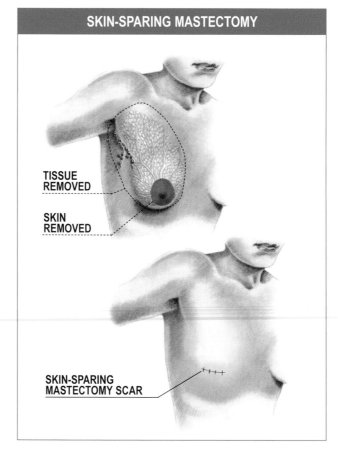

TISSUE REMOVED

SKIN REMOVED

SKIN-SPARING MASTECTOMY SCAR

5. Prophylactic Mastectomy

For some women there may be an option for a prophylactic mastectomy (simple mastectomy) of a breast if bilateral reconstruction is desired. A prophylactic mastectomy takes place before cancer has been found. Some women with an extremely high risk of breast cancer or precancerous conditions in the breast choose this procedure. This elective surgery is a decision made collaboratively between the patient, surgeon and oncologist. A second opinion may be required to ensure that this is a physically and psychologically sound decision. Reasons for considering this procedure may include:

- Family history of breast cancer, including first degree relatives who died of the disease

- Identified carrier of BRCA1 or BRCA2 genes

- Repeated breast biopsies for suspicious findings

- Mammograms that show findings which are increasingly difficult to interpret

- Diagnosis of a cancer type that has a high rate of occurrence in both breasts

- When the weight of a very large remaining breast (after mastectomy) creates imbalance, posture changes and back pain

- Overwhelming psychological fear of occurrence in remaining breast

- Desire for bilateral reconstruction with an increase or decrease in the reconstructed breast size

Lumpectomy Versus Mastectomy

If your breast and tumor are within certain size limits, your surgeon may offer you the option of a lumpectomy (breast conservation) versus a mastectomy. If you are in the category that gives you the option to choose between a lumpectomy and a mastectomy, the decision may be difficult. This needs to be a decision you make in consultation with your physician, after a careful review of the advantages and disadvantages of both. Remember, the option to choose is not available for some types of cancer.

It is imperative that you feel comfortable with the decision. Studies document that a lumpectomy, in an appropriate candidate, even if there is local recurrence, **does not affect survival rate**. However, the inconvenience may come from the necessity to have a second surgery. Ask your surgeon if there are any additional variables in your surgical decision that may be added to this list.

Advantages of Lumpectomy:
- Saves a large portion of the breast, usually the nipple and areola

- Preserves body image

- Allows you to wear your own bras

- Rarely requires reconstruction or the wearing of a prosthesis

- Recovery time from surgery is shorter, usually several weeks

- Slightly shorter hospitalization time or may be performed as outpatient surgery

- May be psychologically easier to accept, unless the fear of monitoring remaining breast tissue for recurrence is too frightening

Disadvantages of Lumpectomy:
- Risk of recurrence of cancer in remaining breast tissue

- Several weeks, usually five to seven, of radiation therapy to the remaining breast tissue

- Changes in texture (lumpiness), color (suntanned appearance) and decreased sensation of feeling in the breast after radiation therapy

- Decrease in size of the remaining breast tissues after swelling decreases following radiation treatments

- Monthly breast self-exam on remaining breast tissue (to monitor for recurrence) becomes more difficult because of increased nodularity (lumpiness) from radiation therapy

- Potential for chronic swelling or accumulation of fluid in the breast (breast lymphedema)

- Possibility of future second lumpectomy or mastectomy if there is a recurrence

Advantages of Mastectomy:

- Removes approximately 95 percent of the breast gland, including the nipple and areola, thus reducing local recurrence to the lowest degree

- Reconstruction of breast is available using your own body tissue or using synthetic implants

Disadvantages of Mastectomy:

- Body image changed because of the removal of a breast

- Need for prosthesis or reconstruction to restore body image

- Recovery time slightly longer than for lumpectomy patients, usually several weeks

If you are having problems making your decision, you may wish to speak with a patient who has already made the choice and had one of the procedures. Ask your physician if there is someone who will be willing to talk to you. Your local American Cancer Society's *Reach to Recovery* program coordinator can provide you with a volunteer's name who will be willing to share her lumpectomy/mastectomy experience.

If you are considering a lumpectomy, you may wish to have a consultation with a radiation oncologist to discuss radiation treatments. Often this consultation will give you additional insight that may help you make a more informed decision. (See Chapter 11 for more information on radiation therapy.)

Refer to Tearout Worksheet
Questions About Surgery - Page 201 & 202
Surgical Decision Evaluation - Page 205 & 206

Second Opinions

When a medical diagnosis is serious and the suggested therapy hard to accept, some women feel the need for additional information or a second opinion. Surgery, chemotherapy and radiation therapy deserve serious consideration, and you need all of the information necessary to make an informed decision. A second opinion is obtained from another physician practicing in the same area of medicine, who reviews your records and offers treatment advice. This opinion may help you feel sure about your treatment decision. **However, for some women, a second opinion may cause anxiety and increase confusion.**

Some insurance providers may require a second opinion before treatment. You will need to check with your insurance provider on this point. Physicians may refer patients for second opinions in order to validate treatment decisions. It is necessary for you to evaluate your needs and decide if a second opinion would be of assistance to you.

Reasons You May Need a Second Opinion:

- You feel insecure or unsure about what you have been told about surgery or treatments.

- Your insurance provider requires a second opinion.

- There has been a disagreement or confusion within your family or with your support partner about the right course of action.

- You want information about newer therapies not offered by your treatment team.

How to Obtain a Second Opinion

If you feel a second opinion would help you resolve your indecisiveness, ask your treatment team for the names of several physicians qualified in this area. Ask the treatment team to list the pros and cons of each one in order to help you determine who will best suit your needs. You may also call a major cancer treatment center for a referral. Some of the national cancer organizations listed in the reference section of this book will give you the names of the major cancer treatment centers located in your area and the services they provide.

Second opinions are often received through pretreatment multidisciplinary conferences held at some centers. A group of physicians from all areas of breast care (radiology, pathology, surgery, medical oncology, radiation oncology, reconstructive surgery) look at your records as a group, discuss your individual case, share their opinions with the group and make treatment recommendations as a team. All of this is done before any of your final treatment decisions are made. This serves as a guide for your own physicians to consider. If you have access to this type of conference, or a group of physicians practicing as a team, this serves as an excellent way to not only have a second opinion, but many expert opinions.

Preparing for the Second Opinion Visit

When seeking a second opinion, you should clarify any questions you have. Make a list of your questions and concerns before the visit and take the list with you. Also, be sure that all requested lab and diagnostic test results are sent to the physician before your visit, to ensure that the needed information is available before the consultation. Call several days prior to your appointment and check to see if your records have arrived. The consulting physician will share his/her opinion with you and send recommendations to your physician, who can then take full advantage of the second opinion.

The most common benefit of a second opinion is to have peace of mind in knowing that you have gathered all the information that you need to make an informed decision. An informed decision allows you to go through your treatments knowing that this was the best treatment choice for you. Some women feel comfortable with their initial treatment options, feel their questions are answered sufficiently and feel no need for a second opinion. This is acceptable for them. Seeking a second opinion is an individual decision and one that needs to be made according to your needs.

REMEMBER

A second opinion is your opportunity to gather all the information you may need to experience peace of mind about your surgical and treatment decisions.

Be sure all your reports are sent prior to your visit and make a written list of all questions you need answered.

Many large centers offer pretreatment multidisciplinary conferences where a team of physicians make recommendations by discussing your case.

If the thought of a second opinion creates anxiety for you, it is not a good idea.

Treatment guidelines for breast cancer can be found from several different sources:
National Comprehensive Cancer Network, www.nccn.org
and American Cancer Society, www.cancer.org

If you insist on seeing with perfect
clearness before you make a decision,
you'll never decide.

The future always looks unclear
like fog; only when you are in the
middle can you see what was
previously hidden from view.

—Judy Kneece

Look at it, size it up, but don't
postpone your life just because
you can't make up your mind.

—Alfred Montapert

Life's problems are like a grindstone;
whether they grind you down or polish
you depends on what you
allow to happen.

—Jacob Braude

RECONSTRUCTIVE SURGERY

"I had immediate reconstruction—a TRAM (used my stomach muscle, skin and fatty tissue to construct a new breast). When I woke up, even though I was bandaged up, I really almost couldn't believe they had removed the breast because the TRAM turned out so well."

—ANNA CLUXTON
SURVIVOR

Even though you are losing a breast or a part of a breast to surgery, you have the option to have your body image restored through plastic surgery. Breast reconstruction has made a big difference, both physically and emotionally, for many women who have undergone surgery for breast cancer. Some have immediate reconstruction at the time of initial breast surgery. They feel that reconstruction will help bring back their feminine silhouette and alleviate the necessity of wearing a prosthesis. Others wait until their treatments for breast cancer have been completed. Some women choose never to have reconstruction.

If you feel that you would like to have your breast reconstructed, talk to your surgeon prior to your surgery. You may also want to consult a reconstructive surgeon prior to your surgery, even if you plan to have the procedure performed after your treatments. Your surgeon or clinic can provide you with names of reconstructive surgeons who have experience in this field.

A decision to have reconstruction requires a lot of research and discussion. Remember, part of gaining control over your cancer is knowing all the options that are available to you and choosing those that best meet your needs.

Types of Reconstruction

There are many types of procedures available today which use implants or your own body tissue to reconstruct your breast. Implants may be filled with saline water or other synthetic material, or with variations of both. Implants are usually placed under your chest muscle. Muscle from your abdomen or back or body fat may also be used to reconstruct your breast. Decisions about which type of surgery would give you the best cosmetic results depend on:

- Your physical makeup (size of your breast, degree of sagging)

- Type of surgery (mastectomy or lumpectomy)

- Treatments given for your cancer (prior radiation therapy to the chest area may not allow some types of reconstruction to be performed)

- Your general health (example: a smoker may be a poor candidate for some types of surgery)

- Your preference for enlargement or reduction of the other breast during surgery

- Your personal goal and motivation for reconstruction. A woman is never too old for reconstructive surgery if she is in good health. Health problems that may cause concern and limit surgical options include:

  - advanced diabetes mellitus

  - recent heart attack or stroke

  - history of severe, chronic lung disease

Only a physician can evaluate the risks for your desired surgical decisions.

Ask your physician or clinic for reconstruction information that explains the surgical procedures and lists all the advantages and disadvantages. The American Cancer Society's *Reach To Recovery* coordinator can give you names of women who have had reconstructive surgery who may be available to discuss their experiences with you.

Reconstruction Reimbursement

In 1998, The Women's Health and Cancer Rights Act (WHCRA) was signed into law providing coverage for women who elect to have a mastectomy to have the cost of reconstruction covered. This law requires insurance providers to cover reconstruction of the surgical breast and surgery, and if needed, to the opposite breast to achieve symmetry (similar shape) between them. It also includes coverage for prostheses and any complications resulting from a mastectomy (including lymphedema, a swelling of the surgical arm).

This law allows women to choose a mastectomy knowing that their reconstruction costs will be covered. If you have any questions or concerns about this law, call the Department of Labor's toll-free number at 1-800-998-7542. You can also call your insurance provider or your State Insurance Commissioner's office. A consultation with a reconstructive surgeon will usually provide the information you need about reimbursement specific to your surgical needs.

Advantages and Disadvantages of Immediate and Delayed Reconstruction

Some of the advantages and disadvantages of immediate and delayed reconstruction are listed below. Ask your reconstructive surgeon for additional comments.

Advantages of Reconstruction:

- Restores feminine body image

- No prosthesis or special bras have to be purchased and worn

- Can wear any clothing, including swimsuits and low-neck attire

- Can go braless for short periods of time, if needed

- Do not have the daily reminder of breast surgery (in the form of a prosthesis)

- Psychologically beneficial in allowing most women to adjust better to the disease

Disadvantages of Reconstruction:

- Physical recovery from surgery will require more time, and you will experience a greater amount of pain

- Increased potential for infection or surgical complications due to the more complex surgery

Immediate Versus Delayed Reconstruction

Advantages of Immediate Reconstruction:

- One surgery experience, requiring anesthesia (being put to sleep) only once

- Lower cost than two separate surgeries

- Reduced recovery time in comparison to two separate surgeries

- Body image does not suffer as great a change as has been associated with mastectomy alone

- Psychologically, there may be some better adaptation

Disadvantages of Immediate Reconstruction:

- More physical discomfort and longer recovery time following surgery, when anxiety levels are at their highest

- Surgery using body tissues requires a much longer surgery and recovery time

- Surgery using implants requires only slightly longer surgery and recovery time

- Increased potential for infection or surgical complications which could delay treatments for your cancer

Advantages of Delayed Reconstruction:

- Time to carefully study reconstruction methods and talk to patients who have experienced varying procedures

- Time to carefully select reconstructive surgeon and seek several consultations if needed

- Psychologically, less anxiety over cancer experience at time of reconstructive surgery

- No delay in treatments (chemotherapy or radiation) because of infection or complications from surgery

- Women who choose delayed reconstruction may be happier with their new breast than women who have immediate reconstruction because they have experienced the inconvenience of having to wear a prosthesis and the inability to go braless (thus their expectations were not as great)

Disadvantages of Delayed Reconstruction:

- Need for a second major surgery

- Higher cost because of second major surgery (anesthesia, surgery room, etc.)

- Cost of purchasing a prosthesis and special bras

- Inconvenience of having to wear a prosthesis until reconstructive surgery

- Temporarily unable to go braless or wear some low-cut clothing

- Procedure may fall into another deductible calendar year, requiring deductibles to be met for a second time (Some insurance providers may not pay for a prosthesis and reconstruction. Only one option for restoring body image may be covered in a policy.)

- Psychological distress from having to deal with an altered body image while waiting on reconstructive surgery

If you are considering reconstruction, make an appointment for a consultation with a plastic surgeon and openly discuss your feelings about the different procedures that may be used. (Questions on page 207) After looking closely at your history, recommended surgical procedure (mastectomy or lumpectomy) and treatment recommendations (chemotherapy or radiation therapy), the surgeon will take into account your desired reconstructive surgery outcome, and a recommendation will be made for you.

Often, women fear that reconstruction may hide or prevent the detection of recurrence of cancer in the breast area. There is no evidence of any kind that breast reconstruction, with your own body tissues or with an implant, causes cancer to grow or recur. Because the breast implant is usually placed beneath the chest wall muscles, there is little difficulty in detecting an early local recurrence. This should not be a concern in making your decision.

Breast Reconstruction Procedures

Breast implants with tissue expanders are the most common type of reconstructive surgery. The procedure may be done immediately, or later as outpatient or inpatient surgery. General anesthesia is usually used and the surgery takes approximately an hour to place the expander under the skin and pectoralis muscle. The expander is gradually filled with a saline (salt water) solution through a valve every few weeks for several months (3 – 6 months) to stretch the muscle and skin before the final implant placement. The skin and muscle are stretched slightly larger than the final implant. Additional surgery is required to remove the expander and position the permanent implant. Some women do not require the tissue expander before implant placement.

TISSUE EXPANDER

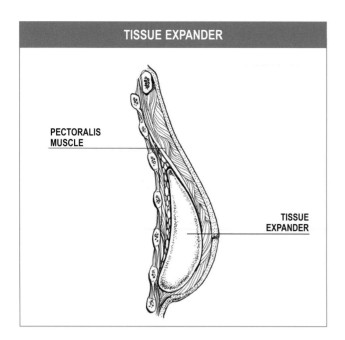

PECTORALIS MUSCLE

TISSUE EXPANDER

Implant (fixed volume implant)

A sack filled with silicone gel or saline fluid is implanted under the skin and chest muscle. Surgery is either outpatient or inpatient and lasts from one to two hours. Local or general anesthesia may be used. Silicone gel implants can be used only in clinical trials. Implants have very few surgical complications. The rates of such common surgical complications as seromas (collection of fluid under skin), hematomas (collection of blood under skin), and infection are relatively low.

Implant Disadvantages:

■ Expander most often requires months to stretch out muscle and skin before body image is restored with implant placement

■ Expander fill-valve may malfunction, requiring replacement

■ Final implant may leak or rupture, requiring replacement

■ Difficult to match a large remaining breast with implants

■ Radiation therapy after implant placement increases risk of complications

■ Capsular contracture risk (tissues around implant harden and distort its shape)

■ Contracture may cause pain, as well as visual change in shape

■ Severe contracture may require removal of implant and placement of new implant

■ Difficult to get reconstructed breast with implant to hang symmetrically on chest wall with opposite breast (implant cannot match natural droop of other breast)

■ Implants will stay same size with weight gain or weight loss, unlike natural breasts

EXPANDER PLACEMENT AND FILLING OF THE EXPANDER

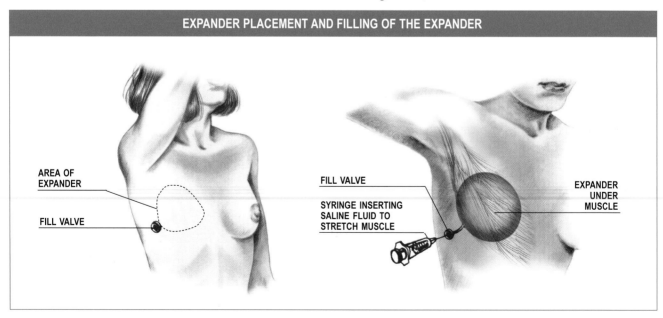

AREA OF EXPANDER

FILL VALVE

FILL VALVE

SYRINGE INSERTING SALINE FLUID TO STRETCH MUSCLE

EXPANDER UNDER MUSCLE

- Implants have a limited lifespan; they deteriorate and need replacement (potentially requiring future surgical procedures)

Indications for Implants:
- Small to medium sized, with no drooping (ptosis)

- No previous radiation therapy to breast area

- Women not wanting additional scars

- Women who do not want longer, more complicated surgery

- Women in poorer general health or advanced age

Autologous (Body Tissues) Reconstruction

Breast reconstruction using a woman's own body tissues (autologous) has many advantages, even with increased surgical complexity. A pedicle flap is a procedure that moves the tissues along with their own blood supply to the area. A free flap procedure cuts the tissues of the selected area from their blood supply and reattaches them through microsurgery to blood vessels in the breast area. Free flaps are the most complex of all reconstructive procedures, requiring a surgeon with expertise in microsurgery.

Advantages:
- Avoids many implant-related complications relating to future surgical procedures for revision or replacement of implant

- Autologous tissues have ample amounts of soft, warm and pliable tissues, more like normal breast tissue, unless a woman is extremely thin

- Normal ptosis (drooping of breast) can be better matched

- Normal inframammary crease (where the wire in an under-wire bra would be positioned) can be better matched to other breast

- Can add additional skin flaps to avoid having to stretch skin if mastectomy scar is tight

- Skin-sparing mastectomy procedure allows immediate reconstruction of the areola, avoiding a later surgical procedure

- Post-surgical deformities or irregularities can be corrected with additional autologous tissues or an autologous flap

- Donor sites (abdomen or hips) can have improvement in contour with reduction of body fat

- Lower cost over time because of fewer future complications and surgical revisions

- Volume and shape of autologous implants follow body weight changes

- Return of breast sensation is possible

- Breast feels warm when touched

- Provides solution for partial mastectomies or wide lumpectomies because of flexibility of tissues

- Preferred reconstruction if radiation therapy is to be part of cancer treatment

The most common sites of autologous tissue retrieval and types of reconstructions are:
- **Abdomen:**
  1. TRAM (transverse rectus abdominis myocutaneous muscle)
  2. DIEP (deep inferior epigastric perforator)*

- **Back:**
  1. LD (latissimus dorsi)
  2. TAP (thoracodorsal artery perforator)*

- **Buttock:**
  1. Free superior or inferior gluteus
  2. S-GAP (free-superior gluteal artery perforator)*

*Perforator flaps
Perforator flaps are recent refinements of conventional flaps where **none** of the underlying muscle is sacrificed. These procedures are relatively new. Ask your healthcare team if your reconstructive surgeons are skilled in these newer techniques.

Advantages of perforator flaps:

- Preserving muscle decreases potential for future problems in donor site (weakness or restriction on activities)

- Preserving underlying muscle allows usual activities of daily living (sports, activities) as before surgery

Disadvantages of perforator flaps (DIEP, TAP, S-GAP):

- Reconstructive surgeon experienced in new procedure is needed

- Prolonged operating time because of complexity of procedure

Abdominal Tissue Reconstruction Procedures

1. TRAM Flap (transverse rectus abdominis myocutaneous muscle)

The transverse rectus abdominis myocutaneous muscle (major stomach muscle) is moved to the breast area with fat and skin and is attached to form a breast. This procedure is most commonly called a tummy tuck. This is the most common type of autologous flap used at present and is excellent for women with additional abdominal fat. The transplanted tissue usually remains connected to its blood supply (called pedicle flap), but occasionally tissues and muscle will be cut loose (free flap) and reconnected by microsurgery. Inpatient surgery is required with general anesthesia, lasting three to five hours and requiring several days of hospitalization. The procedure is moderately painful, causing difficulty in standing up straight for several days or weeks because of the cut muscle. Drains are usually removed after one week, but may be left in place for several weeks. A scar is left on the abdomen where the flap is removed. Disadvantages are an increased weakness of the abdominal muscle and wall, limiting strength and making some activities difficult, along with an increased potential for hernias.

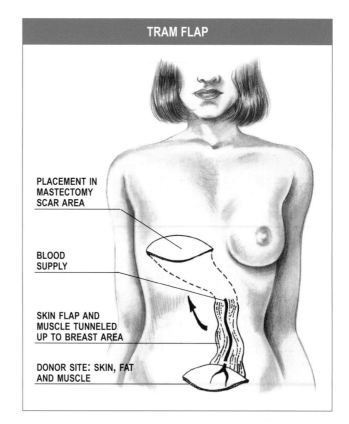

TRAM FLAP

PLACEMENT IN MASTECTOMY SCAR AREA

BLOOD SUPPLY

SKIN FLAP AND MUSCLE TUNNELED UP TO BREAST AREA

DONOR SITE: SKIN, FAT AND MUSCLE

2. DIEP (deep inferior epigastric perforator)

This procedure uses abdominal tissues without the abdominal muscle (rectus abdominis). The fat is harvested with local blood vessels (free flap, cut loose from local blood supply). Nerves can also be harvested along with the flap and used to restore sensation to the tissues when reattached in the breast area. Recovery time is reduced in this procedure compared to the TRAM flap because the muscle is not being moved, allowing earlier mobilization and return to normal activities.

Back Tissue Reconstruction Procedures

1. Latissimus dorsi (back flap)

The back muscle, the latissimus dorsi, along with an eye-shaped wedge of skin are moved from the back and sewn in place on the breast area. The transplanted tissues are left attached to their original blood supply (pedicle flap). This is an inpatient procedure with general anesthesia lasting two to four hours and requires several days of hospitalization. The procedure is moderately painful, and a scar is left on the back. Drains may be left in place for several weeks. An implant, in addition to her own tissue, may be required to match the opposite breast because of the size of the latissimus muscle moved. Some procedures can be performed endoscopically (using special instruments under the skin) without leaving a scar on the back. This procedure is excellent for small, non-drooping breasts or for partial outer quadrant reconstruction.

2. TAP (thoracodorsal artery perforator)

This procedure is an alternative to the latissimus dorsi flap; it does **not** move the muscle, but uses the fat of the upper and lower areas around the muscle. Because some women do not have a lot of additional fat in this area, it may not be the preferred procedure.

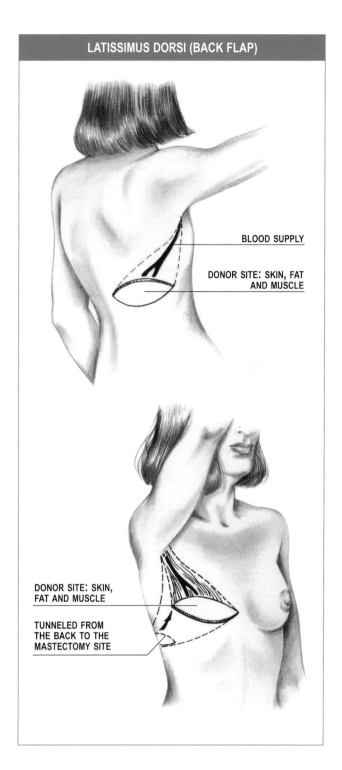

LATISSIMUS DORSI (BACK FLAP)

BLOOD SUPPLY

DONOR SITE: SKIN, FAT AND MUSCLE

DONOR SITE: SKIN, FAT AND MUSCLE

TUNNELED FROM THE BACK TO THE MASTECTOMY SITE

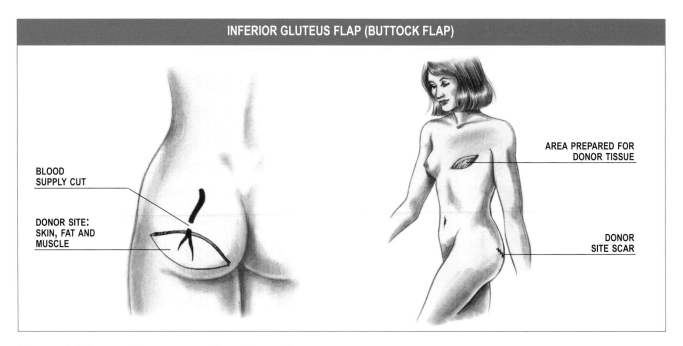

INFERIOR GLUTEUS FLAP (BUTTOCK FLAP)

BLOOD
SUPPLY CUT

DONOR SITE:
SKIN, FAT AND
MUSCLE

AREA PREPARED FOR
DONOR TISSUE

DONOR
SITE SCAR

Buttock Tissue Reconstruction Procedures

1. Inferior (lower) Gluteus (Buttock) Flap

This procedure uses a patient's own tissue from fat and muscle in the buttocks. The tissue is detached (cut free) from its blood supply and reattached to the breast area blood supply using microsurgery. This is an inpatient procedure that includes general anesthesia. Surgery can range from three to eight hours according to the degree of microscopic reattachment necessary. The scars on the buttocks are easily covered with underwear. Most women, except extremely thin ones, have tissue to spare.

2. S-GAP (free-superior gluteal artery perforator)

This is an upgrade of the gluteus flap; it requires **no** muscle to be harvested and only the fatty tissue along with an artery for blood supply are moved to the breast and reattached using microsurgery. The tissue is removed from the upper portion of the buttocks (superior). This area has the potential to remove and transfer nerves to restore sensation to the new breast.

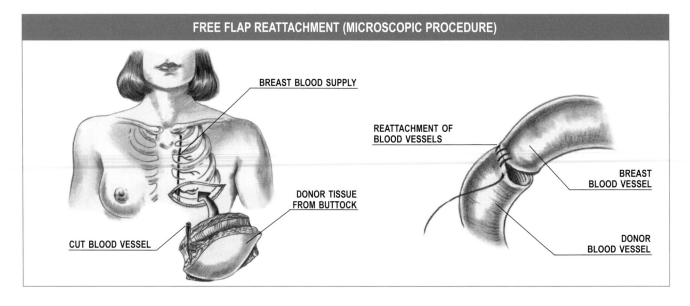

FREE FLAP REATTACHMENT (MICROSCOPIC PROCEDURE)

BREAST BLOOD SUPPLY

REATTACHMENT OF
BLOOD VESSELS

BREAST
BLOOD VESSEL

DONOR TISSUE
FROM BUTTOCK

DONOR
BLOOD VESSEL

CUT BLOOD VESSEL

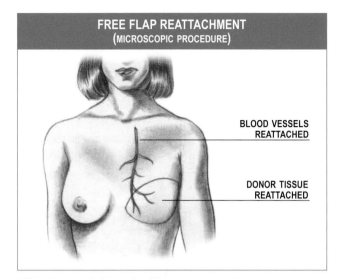

FREE FLAP REATTACHMENT
(MICROSCOPIC PROCEDURE)

BLOOD VESSELS REATTACHED

DONOR TISSUE REATTACHED

Nipple and Areola Reconstruction

The nipple and areola are usually reconstructed from existing skin and fat on the breast itself, or occasionally from tissues removed from other areas of the body such as the groin. The skin is molded to form the shape of the nipple and attached to the breast mound. Areola reconstruction may be done by tattooing a dark pigmented color to match the other areola. Surgery is outpatient and pain is minimal. The procedure is usually performed about six months after reconstruction when breast symmetry is satisfactory. Some women choose not to have their nipple and areola reconstructed after breast reconstructive surgery.

Reconstruction and Breast Cancer Detection

Reconstruction does not alter the biology of breast cancer. It cannot cause an increase in local recurrence and does not compromise the ability to have adequate breast cancer treatment. Women often fear that reconstruction may hide or prevent the detection of cancer recurrence in the breast area in the future. Physicians report, however, that there is little difficulty in detecting early local recurrence because the breast implant is usually placed under the skin and beneath the chest wall muscles. Furthermore, there is no evidence of any kind that breast reconstruction causes cancer to grow or makes it recur. If a woman desires immediate reconstruction, it will not alter her disease-free interval or survival. These fears should not be of any concern in making a decision.

Questions to Ask Your Reconstructive Surgeon:

- What type of surgery do you recommend for me?

- Do you suggest the use of my own body tissue or an implant?

- What kind of implants do you recommend? Will they be placed under the muscle?

- What are the risks and benefits of this surgery?

- Can I see photographs and talk to some of your patients?

- What can I expect to look like after surgery?

- Will you reconstruct my nipple and areola?

- How much feeling (sensation) will I have in my reconstructed breast?

- How will my breast feel when touched (soft, firm)?

- Will this surgery cause me to have additional scars?

- How many surgical procedures will my reconstruction require?

- How long will I be in surgery for each of these procedures?

- How many procedures require hospitalization?

- How many are out-patient procedures?

- How often will I need a return appointment with you?

- How long will it take to complete the reconstruction process?

- How long before I can return to work or normal activities after each procedure?

- How much will it cost, and how much should my insurance cover?

Complications and Risks of Reconstruction Procedures

COMPLICATION RISKS	MUSCLE SPARING (FREE-TRAM OR DIEP)	NON-MUSCLE SPARING	IMPLANTS
Abdominal bulge or hernia	2 - 4%	5 - 10%	
Abdominal weakness	Virtually eliminated	30 - 60%	
Delayed healing	Less than 5% *	Less than 5% *	Less than 5% *
Premature removal related to rupture or capsular contracture or patient dissatisfaction			40% by 5 years
Free flap failure	3%		

*most common with previous radiation or smokers

REMEMBER

Reconstruction is an option that all breast surgery patients need to know about, but not a procedure that all patients necessarily need to have.

Costs of reconstruction for women having a mastectomy are now covered by law. Cost should not be of concern when making your decision.

If all of this information overwhelms you, you do not have to make a decision now. Reconstruction can be performed at a later date, even years later. Make decisions based on what you feel best meets your needs.

Refer to Tearout Worksheets

Questions for Reconstructive Surgeon - Page 207
Reconstructive Surgery Options - Page 208

Comparison of Breast Reconstruction Procedures

TYPE	ADVANTAGES	DISADVANTAGES	INDICATIONS	CONTRAINDICATIONS
Tissue Expander and Implant	■ Short surgical time ■ Low cost	■ Multiple fillings of expander with saline ■ 2nd surgery for implant ■ Capsular contracture ■ Leakage or rupture	■ Medium size breast (400 - 800 cc) ■ Lumpectomy defect ■ Tight skin from radiation therapy	■ None ■ Previous radiation therapy may limit size
Implant: Saline or Silicone	■ Short surgical time ■ One-step procedure ■ Lower cost	■ Capsular contracture ■ Leakage or rupture ■ Autoimmune disease (>.5%)	■ Small breast (400 - 600 cc)	■ Thin skin flaps ■ Radiation therapy
Latissimus Dorsi Flap (Pedicle Flap) **Muscle and Tissue**	■ Autologous tissue and muscle remain attached to blood supply ■ Small donor scar	■ Minor muscle weakness ■ Potential seroma ■ Flap necrosis	■ Small to medium size breast (400 - 800 cc) ■ Lumpectomy defect ■ Tight skin from radiation therapy	■ None
TAP Thoracodorsal Artery Perforator (Free Flap) Tissues Only	■ Autologous tissue with blood vessels ■ No muscle removed ■ Small donor scar	■ Potential seroma ■ Flap necrosis	■ Small to medium sized breast (400 - 800 cc) ■ Lumpectomy defect ■ Tight skin from radiation therapy	■ Extremely thin women
TRAM Flap Transverse Rectus Abdominis Myocutaneous (Pedicle)	■ Autologous muscle with tissues attached to local blood supply ■ Tummy tuck	■ Scar on abdomen ■ Minor muscle weakness ■ Extended operative time ■ 6 - 12 wks. recovery ■ Abdominal wall hernia ■ Flap necrosis	■ Mastectomy	■ Previous abdominal surgery ■ Physical condition ■ Cigarette smokers (some physicians)
DIEP Deep Interior Epigastric Perforator (Free Flap)	■ Abdominal tissues with blood vessels and nerves ■ Potential return of nerve sensations in area	■ Additional scar on abdomen ■ Extended operative time from microscopic reattachment ■ Flap necrosis	■ Mastectomy	■ Previous abdominal surgery ■ Physical condition ■ Cigarette smokers (some physicians) ■ Extremely thin women
Inferior Gluteus Flap (Free Flap)	■ Autologous tissues, muscle and blood vessels cut from lower buttocks	■ Scar at donor site ■ 6 - 12 weeks recovery ■ Extended surgical reattachment time ■ Flap necrosis	■ Mastectomy	■ Cigarette smokers (some physicians) ■ Extremely thin women
S-GAP Superior Gluteal Artery Perforator (Free Flap)	■ Autologous tissues, blood vessels, and nerves cut from upper buttocks ■ Potential return of nerve sensation	■ Scar at donor site ■ Shorter recovery ■ Extended surgical reattachment time ■ Flap necrosis	■ Mastectomy	■ Cigarette smokers (some physicians) ■ Extremely thin women

Life has its hurts, pains and
disappointments for everyone and
is part of the human experience.
Expecting losses and disappointments
as a normal part of life keeps us from
being overwhelmed when they occur.
The secret is to take your hurts, pains
and disappointments and use them to
learn how to build a better life.
Since you can't avoid them,
learn to use them as tools for
refining and redesigning
your life.

—Judy Kneece

Going through loss and grief is like
going through a tunnel.
The bad news is the tunnel is dark.
The good news is once you have
entered into that tunnel,
you're already on
your way out.

—Dr. Robert Jeffress

THE SURGICAL EXPERIENCE

"I had the normal fear of adjusting to the loss of my breast, but by now I was more angry than afraid. My worst nightmare had become a reality."

—HARRIETT BARRINEAU
SURVIVOR

"Probably the most alone I have ever felt was the five minutes after my husband left my side before I went into surgery. Alone, scared of the unknown, so afraid. I felt like my heart was going to beat out of my chest. But then the anesthesia took effect and I went to sleep, and what seemed like minutes later, my surgeon was waking me up. In reality it was 8 hours later! Brian also says this was the hardest time for him."

—ANNA CLUXTON
SURVIVOR

Prior to your surgery you will need to have a pre-admission physical assessment that is usually performed in the hospital where your surgery will take place. Lab work includes a profile of your blood components and body chemistry, urinalysis, chest x-ray, electrocardiogram and any other tests your physician may feel are necessary. **Remember to take your insurance card or policy when going for this assessment**. If you have a living will or any special instructions, take them with you to be attached to your chart the day of surgery. It is now customary for everyone entering a hospital to be asked if they have a living will before any admission. This is asked of all patients and has nothing to do with your type of treatment or diagnosis. Also, take a list of any medications, prescription or non-prescription, that you regularly take. This also includes all herbal products that you are taking.

A registered nurse will conduct an interview asking questions about your physical and medical history. You will be asked dates of previous surgeries or major illnesses and to list any allergies that you have experienced. Don't dismiss any detail as too insignificant or embarrassing to mention. It is better that the medical team be aware than be surprised by some complication. Tell the nurse or physician if you are under the care of another specialist, such as a cardiologist or pulmonologist, prior to your surgery. Be sure that your surgeon is aware of their names and telephone numbers. This assessment usually takes one to two hours.

You will be given instructions about any special preparations before surgery. For example, you will be told not to eat or drink after midnight the day of your surgery and to stop smoking as early before surgery as possible. **Ask the nurse if you should take any of your regular medications the morning of surgery**. The time you should arrive before your surgery and the scheduled time of your surgery will be provided during your pre-admission visit. Ask if there are any restrictions on the number of people allowed to wait in the surgical waiting room. Ask if cell phones are allowed in the waiting room. Request the telephone number to this waiting room to provide for other family members or friends.

Blood transfusions are rarely needed with lumpectomy and mastectomy surgeries. Occasionally, some types of reconstruction may require that blood be available if needed. Your reconstructive surgeon will inform you if your type of surgery may possibly need to have blood available. Information on how to arrange to have your blood collected and stored can be provided by your doctor.

Packing for Overnight Hospital Visit

When packing your suitcase to take to the hospital for an overnight stay, you will need to remember:

- Personal hygiene items: comb, brush, toothbrush, toothpaste, deodorant, makeup and shampoo

- Robe and gown or pajamas (two to three changes—better if they are front-opening)

- Undergarments

- Bedroom shoes

- Reading material

- Telephone numbers of family and friends

- Pencil and note paper

- Pillow to elevate your arm in hospital and to use with your seatbelt on your ride home

- Clothes to wear home. Some women find that large, soft sweatshirts or loose-fitting, front-opening tops are comfortable. Flat, comfortable shoes are recommended.

- Some surgeons and reconstructive surgeons place a special post-operative surgical bra on a patient immediately after surgery. Ask your surgeon if they use surgical bras. If not, you may wish to be prepared by talking to your surgeon about recommendations.

- Lumpectomy patients need to ask their surgeon about recommendations for a well-fitting, soft, front closing bra to wear after surgery. It is recommended that you purchase two or more before surgery to have another available if one gets soiled or wet.

- Mastectomy patients need to ask the surgeon about recommendations for a bra and how to restore your body image if you have a mastectomy without reconstruction. Local prosthetic stores have soft fiber puffs that will fill the surgical side of the bra cup until you are healed and can purchase a prosthesis. You don't have to wear a bra; this is a decision for women who want their body image restored as soon as possible. Many women choose to obtain this before surgery so that the fiber puff can be matched to the size of their breast.

- Reconstructive patients need to ask the surgeon for recommendations on prior purchase of a special type of bra to wear after surgery.

Outpatient Surgery Preparation:

- To surgery, wear loose-fitting, front-opening, comfortable clothing along with comfortable shoes that are suitable for your return home.

- Pack a bag with a comb or brush, mirror, toothbrush and toothpaste.

- Take a bra to wear after surgery as discussed above.

It will be psychologically and physically helpful to have someone plan to be with you on the day of surgery. A trained nurse is not necessary because mastectomy and lumpectomy surgeries are usually relatively simple and do not involve extensive assistance after surgery. A family member or friend will be able to assist you and make this time more comfortable (for example, by helping you to the bathroom or getting you something to drink).

Informed Consent

Sometime before your surgery you will be asked to sign an informed consent form. Consent forms will also be presented before chemotherapy, radiation therapy or reconstructive surgery for your signature.

Your physician or an assistant will explain the procedures that will be performed and the possible risks involved. This will occur before sedation is given. Read the consent form carefully. It will contain the following information:

- Type of surgery and treatment you will receive

- Name of the doctor who will perform the surgery or treatment

- Risks of the surgery or treatment

- Advantages of the surgery or treatment

- Identification of any experimental treatments

- Benefits of the surgery or treatment

- When the treatment will begin and end

By signing this form you acknowledge that you understand and have no other questions. Discuss with the surgeon what type of post-operative pain management will be used and if the medication will be given on request. If you do not understand and would like more information, this is the time to request it.

The Day of Your Surgery

On the day of surgery you will need to report to the surgery area at the assigned time. Do not wear jewelry (watches, rings, earrings) or contact lenses. Eyeglasses may be needed to read and sign admission forms. Dental bridges or false teeth can be worn and removed just prior to your surgery. The nurse will place them in a special storage container during surgery and they will be made available to you as soon as you are alert. Do not bring money, credit cards or a checkbook. Leave these with family members or at home.

You will be interviewed by your anesthesiologist (the physician who administers the anesthesia) before going to surgery. Some anesthesiologists may prefer an interview prior to the day of surgery. Your medical history will be reviewed before surgery. Inform your nurse if any changes in your health have occurred since the initial assessment (cold, fever, diarrhea, etc.).

You will be taken to a room where you will undress and begin preparing for surgery. You will be given a medication to keep you calm. Your underarm area will be shaved. An intravenous needle to be used for medications and fluids will be inserted into the arm opposite the surgical site.

After entering the surgical suite you will be positioned upon a surgical table. A cuff will be placed on your arm to monitor your blood pressure, a device will be placed on your finger to measure the oxygen in your blood, and an electrocardiogram machine will be hooked up to monitor your heart. The surgeon will cleanse a large area surrounding the site of the surgical incision. You will be given your anesthesia some time during this process. After you are asleep, you will have a tube placed in your throat to facilitate your breathing. Your surgery will then be performed.

When the surgical procedure is completed you will be transferred to a post-anesthesia (recovery) room. Your blood pressure, oxygen level and heart rate will be monitored while in this room. Usually, you are in recovery for two or more hours according to the type of anesthesia you received. When you are awake and your vital signs are in normal range, you will be transferred to your room or allowed to return home if you are having outpatient surgery. Your family members will be able to join you at this time. If you are to leave the same day, you may be transferred to an outpatient recovery room and monitored for several more hours before being dismissed.

If staying in the hospital, your blood pressure, pulse and respirations will be monitored at regular intervals. You will have a bandage on your chest and may have one or more bulb drains to avoid fluid collection in the surgical site. Some lumpectomies may not require a drain. At first the drainage will be bright red from blood, but it will gradually change color over the next few days. If at any time you notice that your bandage feels wet or you see bright red blood coming through your bandage, notify your healthcare team. These drain(s) may remain in place after you return home. However, sometimes the physician may remove the drain before you leave the hospital.

Discomfort After Surgery

Most women are surprised at the small amount of pain they experience after their surgery. Pain medication has been ordered by the physician to control any pain you experience. If an inpatient, you must request it from the nurse. If you have pain, use your nurse call button to let your nurse know so the medication can be administered. If you return home, take the prescribed pain medication as ordered.

The pain experienced after breast surgery has been described by women as a discomfort in the breast area, accompanied with numbness or tingling in the arm. Others say that they felt pain in the removed breast that felt like a heaviness or sensations from the nipple. Doctors call this **phantom pain** because even though the breast is gone, the brain perceives the sensation of pain from the remaining nerves. Some of the nerves on the chest wall may be irritated or cut during the surgical procedure, and this causes a feeling of numbness across the chest. Most women state that most discomfort is under the arm where the lymph nodes were removed. This pain often radiates down the arm, and you may feel as if needles or pins are pricking you. The arm may also feel numb. The numbness is not unusual, and the sensation may or may not improve in the coming months. Incisional pain is usually over in about a week to ten days, and the referred sensations will improve as arm mobility is restored. The surgical staff's goal is that you experience the minimum amount of pain, and they will provide you with the amount of medication required to keep you comfortable.

After you wake up, you may also have a slight headache or nausea from the residual anesthesia. This is not unusual and often may be caused from the long period of time you have been without food. Resume eating by taking fluids first, add light foods and then progress to your normal diet as you desire. Nausea can be increased by heavy foods.

Your throat may feel sore from the tube inserted during surgery. Soreness in the back or shoulder area is very common because of the position you were required to be in during surgery. This soreness will last for several days.

Personal Hygiene After Surgery

For the next few days you may need to take a sponge bath to keep your dressing dry. Ask your doctor when you have permission for a shower or a tub bath. The dressing should always be kept dry. If at any time the dressing becomes wet, you need to have it changed. Dressings that are damp and remain over the incision can cause a local infection.

Your physician will tell you when you can use your surgical arm to shampoo your hair. Do not use deodorant under the surgical arm for the first six weeks. Perspiration odor is unusual because of glands removed during surgery. However, you may wipe the area with an alcohol pad or peroxide if you feel a need to cleanse the area. Avoid allowing the alcohol to run into the surgical area and cause stinging.

Post-Surgical Arm Care

Your surgical arm will be sore but you need to continue to use your hand to feed yourself, comb your hair and wash your face. This will help the soreness to improve. Keeping your surgical arm propped up on a pillow, above the level of your heart, will assist in preventing fluid accumulation and swelling in the arm, reducing the pain. It is helpful if you can elevate your arm for 45 minutes, twice a day for the first six weeks after surgery. But **do not lift** anything heavy (over 1-2 pounds) or **begin any exercises** until your **physician gives you permission**. It is also helpful to keep the arm from pressing tightly against the body after surgery. This reduces the ability of the fluid accumulation from surgery to drain from the area. Using a small pillow between the arm and body will keep the arm in a position that promotes drainage and reduces swelling.

Rest After Surgery

The time spent in the hospital will be only a day or a few days. During this time you may feel sleepy and tired from the anesthesia and all the stress that accumulated prior to the surgery. If you don't feel up to having many visitors, ask your nurse to place a "No Visitors" sign on your door. If you return home the same day of surgery, you may also want to have your family members monitor visitors so that you can get the amount of rest you need.

You may also take the telephone off the hook or turn the ringer off when you are trying to rest. Ask family members or friends to speak to visitors or answer the telephone if you feel you need rest. Remember to ask for or take medications to keep you comfortable. If hospitalized, pain and nausea medications have to be requested by the patient.

The Surgical Incision

Your first dressing change will occur before you leave the hospital unless you have outpatient surgery—in which case, you will return to the physician's office. Some women report it was difficult to view the incision for the first time, but afterwards they were glad they did. Viewing the incision may also be difficult for your mate. Many women feel that viewing the incision together the first time was helpful in their future adjustment. Postponing the viewing does not make it easier or help either of you.

It is important that you observe the incision area carefully at this time to learn what is normal for the scar area. This will help as you monitor the incision for changes after you return home. A mastectomy scar is one long scar. You may have sutures or staples to close the incision. A lumpectomy will have an incision on the breast and another under the arm if lymph nodes were removed. Your doctor or nurse will provide instructions at this time on how and when to change the dressing and changes to report to the medical staff. It will be helpful if a family member is present during these instructions to help you understand and be able to assist you with dressing changes and managing drains.

Care of Your Dressing

The goal of care for your incision is to keep a clean, dry dressing in place and monitor the area for changes that might indicate an infection. Types of dressings vary with physicians, but all dressings need to remain dry. A wet dressing will set up an environment for bacteria to breed and may cause an infection. If your dressing becomes damp, follow your physician's instructions

for changing it. Sutures or staples are removed five to ten days later in the doctor's office.

Your surgeon or nurse will discuss care of your dressing prior to discharge. It may help to have a family member assist with dressing changes because of the soreness you will experience and the difficulty of working on your own chest. It is helpful if they are present when dressing changes are discussed. Ask your nurse for dressing supplies to take home. Follow special orders from your physician for dressing changes. If you do not receive orders, the steps to follow for changing a dressing are listed below.

Dressing Change Instructions

1. Gather all dressing supplies: paper bag, dressing (gauze), tape, scissors, alcohol wipes or gauze pads

2. Wash your hands

3. Pre-cut tape into strips to apply to new dressing

4. Remove the old dressing

5. Note the color, odor and amount of drainage on dressing

6. Dispose of the old dressing in a paper bag

7. Wash your hands thoroughly with soap

8. Observe incision carefully

9. Wipe off any old blood or tape residue with an alcohol wipe. Always start wiping near the incision and wipe away from the incision, not back over it.

10. Place clean dressing on the area and tape it into place

11. Dispose of paper bag containing old dressing and alcohol wipes

12. Wash your hands

Monitoring Your Incision

When changing your dressing, observe the old bandage for signs of drainage. Normal drainage is a blood-tinged, watery discharge. Discharge that is thick and yellowish to greenish in color may indicate infection. Often this type of discharge will have a foul odor. If you notice this occurring, notify your health-care provider.

Carefully observe the incision site. An increase in redness, swelling and signs of discharge anywhere along the incision line may indicate a potential infection. Call your physician's office and ask for instructions. Often, early intervention may require a local antibiotic to the area.

Ask your physician when you may take a shower or tub bath and use soap and water on the area. Some physicians allow showers first because of the constant flow of clean water over the incision. After your bath/shower, pat the area dry and protect it with a soft dressing or covering to prevent irritation and rubbing by your clothing. Some find that a soft tee shirt or a long-line cotton sports bra, which is sold in department stores, serves this purpose.

It is important to not allow any powder, deodorant, lotions or perfumes to come in contact with the surgical incision site. These products should be avoided for four to six weeks past surgery or until the site has healed completely. You may wipe the area with an alcohol wipe or peroxide to further cleanse after your bath.

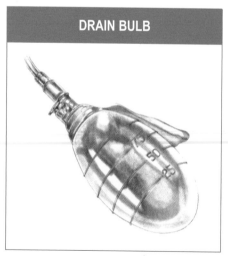

DRAIN BULB

Care of Your Drain Bulbs

Instructions will also be given on how to care for your drain(s) if you have them. Drains are inserted to collect fluid accumulation at the surgery site and to reduce swelling and pain. The tubing is anchored to your tissue during surgery. At the end of the tubing is a soft plastic bulb with a plug that allows the fluid to be emptied.

The fluid that accumulates in the drain bulb is a mixture of blood cells and lymphatic fluid. During surgery, the lymphatic system vessels are cut, causing the microscopic vessels to empty their fluid into the area. The drainage will be dark red at first because of the large amount of blood cells in the area. It will gradually change to pink-tinged and finally to a yellow, straw color. The amount of drainage varies, and there is no way to predict how much drainage any woman will accumulate. Some women have large amounts and others have a minimal amount. Gradually, these small vessels seal themselves off, and the fluid stops accumulating. The time this takes varies among women. Neither body size nor age seems to determine the amount; however, the amount of drainage during the first 24 hours often predicts the accumulation volume later.

Physicians remove the drains when the amount of drainage is reduced to between 20 to 50 ccs (½ to 1 ½ ounces or 4 to 10 teaspoons) per drain, per 24 hours. Some women have very little drainage and have their drain(s) removed within the first week. Others may need their drain(s) for several weeks and, occasionally, longer. If the drain(s) are removed too soon, the fluid can accumulate under the skin, forming a seroma (collection of fluid), and become painful by putting pressure on the surgical site. Neither the amount of fluid produced nor the length of time required to have drains has anything to do with your cancer. Fluid and drains are only related to the amount of fluid your lymph system produces.

Care of your drains will be discussed by your nurse. It is important not to allow the drains to hang loosely. **Always secure them to your clothing and empty them when they become heavy.** The first day may require emptying every several hours. Later, twice a day will be sufficient. Pressure caused from a heavy drain, not pinned to your clothing and pulling on your incision site, can cause **pain and scar formation at the drain insertion site**. The scar will heal but will be thick and have an uneven appearance. Be careful not to allow drains to drop away from your body.

Emptying and Recording Your Drainage

Empty drains when they become heavy or over half-filled with fluid. When your drainage has decreased to a small amount, empty twice a day.

1. If you have more than one drain, place a piece of tape on each, and mark them with numbers (drain 1 or drain 2). Refer to the amounts emptied, and record by number designation.

2. Gather your supplies: a drain record (found on page 213), pencil or pen and a measuring cup.

3. Open one drain by removing the plug in the drain bulb, and empty drainage into a measuring cup.

4. Squeeze the air out of the empty bulb and keep the bulb squeezed as flat as possible as you replug the drain. This compression of the bulb encourages the flow of fluid from the surgical site into the bulb.

5. If any of the drainage spilled onto the outside of the bulb, wipe it off with a damp cloth using soap and water or an alcohol wipe.

6. Secure the bulb by pinning it to your clothing or placing it into a surgical drainage bag holder. Do not allow the bulb to hang freely.

7. Measure the drainage in the cup.

8. Observe the color of the drainage. If you begin noticing that the fluid has changed color, becoming a darker red or fresh blood reappearing after the color had changed to a light pink, contact your physician's office and inform them of the change.

9. Empty the drainage into the toilet and flush. You do not save the drainage.

10. Wash your hands with soap and water.

11. Record drainage under the appropriate column, documenting the time and amount emptied.

12. If you have a second drain, repeat the process.

13. Take the written drainage record to the surgeon on your return visit. An accurate record will assist the physician in determining when to remove your drain(s). (A tearout worksheet to record your drainage at home is located on page 213 of this workbook.)

Potential Post-Surgical Problems

Fluid Leakage at Drain Site

Occasionally, a small amount of fluid will leak from the insertion site of the tubing. This is not dangerous. However, you should apply a sterile dressing and change the dressing when it becomes damp. Do not allow a wet dressing to remain in place. The dressing should be changed as often as needed to prevent irritation and breakdown of the skin. A wet dressing will allow bacteria to grow. If large amounts of fluid begin leaking from the site, call your surgeon or nurse and ask for instructions.

Clogged Drains

Bulb drains may clog because of the formation of small clots in the tubing. This is not an unusual occurrence. If you notice that there is no fluid in the bulb, check the tubing for a possible blockage caused by a clot. If a clot is found or if your drain has stopped draining, perform the following steps to reopen drainage:

1. Wash your hands with soap and water.

2. Gently squeeze the area in which the clot is located to dislodge it.

3. After squeezing the clot, begin near the insertion site on your chest and squeeze downward the entire length of the tubing toward the drainage bulb. Do not pull on the tubing. Repeat the process several times, squeezing the entire length of the drainage tubing.

4. Secure drains to prevent hanging loosely.

5. Monitor the drain bulb for fluid accumulation. If no drainage has accumulated after several hours, notify your physician for further instructions.

Monitoring Drains for Infection

It is very rare for infections to occur with bulb drains. However, if you notice the insertion site begins to have an increased redness, discharge of pus (thick yellowish or greenish fluid) or foul odor, then notify your physician of these changes. The main prevention for infection is to keep the area clean and dry.

Drain Removal

Drains are removed by the surgeon or an assistant during an office visit. Women report a pulling feeling with a moderate amount of pain lasting for a few seconds when the drain is removed. A small bandage is placed over the drain removal site. This site will also need to be monitored for infection for the next several days. Any increase in redness, swelling, discharge or pain should be reported to your surgeon's office.

Seromas

Before or after your drains are removed, if you have a painful accumulation of fluid at the incision site, below the incision site or in the underarm area, notify your physician. This fluid accumulation is called a **seroma**. The accumulation of fluid feels much like water in a balloon when it forms under the skin. If a seroma continues to increase in size and puts pressure on your incision, it can become painful.

Seromas are the most common complication after surgery. Painful seromas may require the withdrawal of the fluid from the area using a small needle and an empty syringe by the physician. This procedure is performed in the physician's office. Withdrawal of the fluid is relatively painless, and removal of the fluid relieves the pain. However, as with any invasive procedure, the potential for infection increases. You will need to monitor the area and report any redness, swelling or pain to your physician. Occasionally, the fluid will continue to accumulate, requiring several

aspirations by the surgeon. This fluid accumulation has nothing to do with your cancer. It is related only to lymphatic fluid accumulation in the area.

Hospital Discharge Instructions

Prior to leaving the hospital or surgical center, your nurse will provide you with verbal and written instructions concerning your care and a list of symptoms that might occur and need to be reported to the doctor. Write down any questions as they occur. Clarify the following with your physician:

- If you do not remember what you were told about your surgery or diagnosis, ask for clarification.

- What activities can I do with my surgical arm until my next appointment?

- Are there any special exercises or recommendations regarding use of my arm?

- Are the numbness or tingling sensations I am experiencing temporary or permanent?

- What kind of pain is normal after my type of surgery?

- What medications will I take for pain?

- Will I be given any prescriptions for medication to take home?

- Do I resume previous medications (especially estrogen-type medications)?

- When can I shampoo my hair?

- When can I shower or take a tub bath?

- When can I remove my bandage?

- When can I drive?

- When and how do I make my next appointment?

- Will I be referred to any other doctors or have any other treatments? If so, when will I see these doctors?

- When will my final pathology report be available?

- Is there anything special that I can do to ensure a speedy recovery?

Ask your nurse to write down any appointment dates or names of doctors to whom you will be referred for further evaluation concerning treatment. Inform your doctor or nurse early if you have a physical limitation that would prevent you from being able to manage at home. A home health service or aide who will assist you for a short period of time can be ordered before you leave the hospital. Ask for a telephone number that you can call after you return home if you have any questions regarding your discharge instructions. Some hospitals will provide you with supplies necessary for your dressing changes at home. Ask your nurse about dressing supplies. (Discharge questions on page 215)

Seatbelt Use After Surgery

On your ride home after surgery it will be helpful if you have a small pillow to place over your chest and the area of your incision so that you will be able to wear your seat belt in the car. Sudden stops can cause pain and potential injury to new mastectomy or lumpectomy surgical sites from the sudden pressure of a seat belt. The protection provided by the pillow can prevent this type of injury or discomfort and make the wearing of your seat belt more comfortable. Using the pillow for protection when wearing a seat belt is helpful for the first several weeks after your surgery if the seat belt crosses your incision.

Recovering at Home

Your discharge instructions from the hospital give you information as to when you need to call the physician, how to manage your drains and how to change your bandage. Recovery from surgery for breast cancer usually requires two to three weeks. Discomfort in the incisional area(s) will improve daily, usually resolving within ten days. In five to six weeks most women report that they have resumed their normal activities. Remember, we are all different. Listen to the cues from your body, rest when needed and resume your normal activities when you feel up to them.

Your incision will change color as it heals; this is normal. Initially the scar will be red and raised for several months past surgery. The redness is caused by the additional blood flow to promote healing in the area. The redness and thickness of the scar will subside over the next one to two years, and the area will become less obvious and very faint in color.

Plan to begin your exercise program to restore your normal range of motion to the surgical arm as soon as the physician gives you permission. Report any problems you have when performing the exercises to your physician.

It is important that you keep your follow-up appointments with the surgeon and any other physicians. You will be monitored for proper healing and the return of proper range of motion in your surgical arm. Your remaining breast will also be closely checked on following visits.

Uncommon Post-Surgical Problems

Most women have very few problems after breast surgery. However, there are some uncommon problems that may arise from the surgical procedure that you may need to be aware of. These problems have nothing to do with the cancer and are only due to the surgery.

Phlebitis

Occasionally some women will have very little pain after their surgery only to experience a pain that begins days after surgery. The pain may radiate down the arm, usually to the elbow, but sometimes to the wrist. This occurs when the basilic vein in the arm has become inflamed after the surgery. This inflammation, called phlebitis, is not serious; it causes pain that can be helped with an analgesic such as aspirin or ibuprofen. Phlebitis is not a common occurrence and will resolve in several days to a week. This pain may limit your ability to perform your exercises. Inform your physician if this should occur.

Sensitive Surgical Site

Another problem a very small percent of women experience is sensitive skin in the surgical area. After surgery, even clothing is painful if it touches the incision area. If this occurs, inform your physician. Occasionally, the nerves in the area are super sensitive and will need a procedure called "desensitization" to decrease the sensation. This procedure is performed by a physical therapist. The therapist can instruct you on the procedure to perform at home if needed, and this then becomes part of your daily exercise routine.

Frozen Shoulder

Failure to use your arm after the physician has given you permission to begin exercises to restore normal range of motion can result in a condition called a "frozen shoulder." This condition causes pain and inability to move the shoulder freely; however, it is a rare occurrence. Any complication that can keep you from proceeding with your exercise program should be brought to the surgeon's attention. Restoring full range of motion is accomplished by gradually increasing the movements of the arm and using exercises such as the ones in Chapter 18.

Refer to Tearout Worksheets
Drain Bulb Record - Page 213
Hospital Discharge Instructions - 215

REMEMBER

Surgery for breast cancer is usually not very physically painful, but it may be very emotionally painful.

Ask your healthcare team for what you need to make this time as easy as possible for you; additional information or instructions, pain medication, privacy, access to a chaplain, etc. You are employing them to meet your needs.

Tell your support partner, family or friends what you need from them during this time. Be honest.

Do not hesitate to call your physician if any problems arise when you return home.

Use the time of your surgery to rekindle your emotions and energy. Rest when needed. Be good to yourself. Think about any changes you would like to make in your life. At no other time in life will people give you as much permission to make changes.

What is it you have always wanted to do—a new hobby, go on a trip, take a class, get a pet, or start an exercise program? You decide what will give you the most happiness and GO FOR IT.

Breast cancer is not a valid excuse to forego planning for events and activities that will bring you happiness. Plan your exciting new future! Use breast cancer as the reason and not the excuse!

UNDERSTANDING YOUR PATHOLOGY REPORT

"I was serious about wanting to know about breast cancer. I wanted to be a part of my treatments. I wanted to know what was being done and why. The secrets to my individual tumor lay in my final pathology report."

—HARRIETT BARRINEAU
SURVIVOR

The preliminary pathology report you received after your biopsy contained much information about your cancer. A final pathology report will be prepared after your surgery that will give additional information about your cancer and the status of cancer in your lymph nodes. Your treatment plan is based on both the preliminary and the final pathology reports. From this series of reports your physicians will determine which course of treatment is best suited for your individual case. The most common treatments are surgery, chemotherapy, radiation therapy and hormonal therapy. Your treatment may consist of one or more types of treatment. For some women, no further treatment may be needed, only close observation by the physician. A brief explanation of each type of treatment will be discussed. Because of the wide variety of treatment plans, your physician will provide you with specific information regarding your planned treatment.

Your Pathology Report

Because treatment decisions will be based on the pathology reports on your tumor, it may be helpful to understand its importance in determining your treatment options. However, it is **not** essential that you understand all of the following information. Some people feel that this is more information than they want to know. Feel free to skip this section. It is included in case you need to have some questions about your pathology report clarified.

After your tumor was removed from your breast, it was sent to a pathology laboratory. There, a pathologist (a physician who specializes in diagnosing diseases from tissue samples) analyzed your tissues under a microscope and issued a pathology report to your physician. This report contains the unique characteristics of your individual tumor. This report will help your physicians determine if you need additional treatment. If additional treatment is needed, the pathology report will be used as a guide for all of your physicians to develop a treatment plan for your cancer.

The slides and tissue blocks prepared by the pathologist to study your tumor and interpreted in your pathology report remain available for additional consults and future studies if future research unfolds with new tissue diagnostic tests.

Characteristics of Cancer Cells

- **Normal Cells**—Normal ducts and lobules are lined with one or more layers of cells in an orderly pattern.

- **In Situ Cancer**—It is called "in situ cancer" when these normal cells become abnormal and cancer develops and grows. In situ cancer does not break through the wall but remains in the duct or lobule where it began. This type has a good prognosis.

- **Invasive (Infiltrating) Cancer**—Cancers that have broken through the wall of the duct or lobule and have begun to grow into surrounding tissues in the breast are considered invasive or infiltrating cancers. "Microinvasive" means just a small amount of cells have grown through the cells walls.

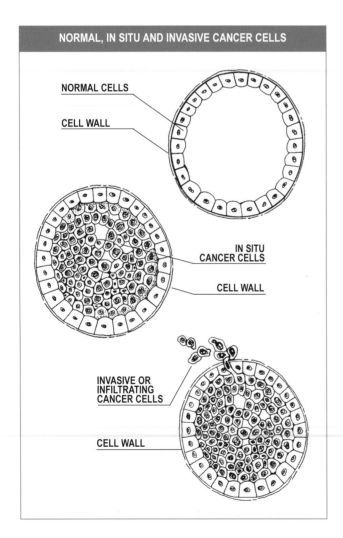

NORMAL, IN SITU AND INVASIVE CANCER CELLS

NORMAL CELLS

CELL WALL

IN SITU CANCER CELLS

CELL WALL

INVASIVE OR INFILTRATING CANCER CELLS

CELL WALL

Types of Breast Cancer

The most common types of breast cancer are listed below. There are also various other rare types of breast cancer and combinations of the following types.

- Infiltrating (invasive) ductal (approximately 52% of patients)

- In situ ductal (intraductal) (approximately 21%)

- Invasive lobular (approximately 5%)

- In situ lobular (intralobular) (approximately 2%)

- Medullary (approximately 6%)

- Mucinous or colloid (approximately 3%)

- Paget's disease with intraductal (approximately 1%)

- Paget's disease with invasive ductal (approximately 1%)

The remaining cancers occur in 1% or less:

- Tubular
- Cribiform
- Papillary
- Micropapillary
- Apocrine
- Adenocystic
- Inflammatory
- Carcinosarcoma
- Squamous

Tumor Size

Tumor size is the measured size of the tumor. Results are reported in millimeters (mm) or centimeters (cm).

- 10 mm equals 1 cm

- 1 cm equals 3/8 inch

- 1 inch equals 2.5 cm

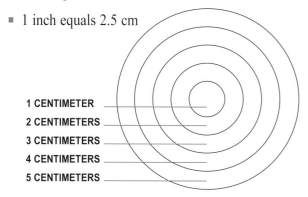

1 CENTIMETER
2 CENTIMETERS
3 CENTIMETERS
4 CENTIMETERS
5 CENTIMETERS

Tumor Shape

The report may also state the shape of a solid tumor as being round, spherical or having irregular contour such as stellate or spiculated.

Margins

Margins are the area cut by the surgeon's knife surrounding your tumor. If the surrounding tissue or breast had no evidence of cancer cells then the terms used will be "negative," "clear," "clean" or "uninvolved." If cancer is found in the margins, the terms maybe "positive," "involved" or "residual cancer." If the pathologist could not determine and make a definite statement the term used may be "indeterminate."

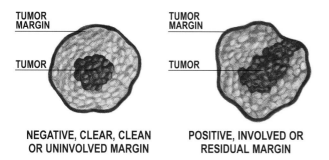

NEGATIVE, CLEAR, CLEAN
OR UNINVOLVED MARGIN

POSITIVE, INVOLVED OR
RESIDUAL MARGIN

Node Status

If surgery included lymph node removal using sentinel node or axillary dissection, the report will state how many nodes were removed, a description of the area from which nodes came and how many nodes tested positive with cancer cells.

Nuclear Grade

An evaluation of the size and shape of the nucleus in tumor cells and the percentage of tumor cells that are in the process of dividing or growing. Cancers with a low nuclear grade grow and spread less quickly than cancers with a high nuclear grade.

Grading of Tumor

The general grading of cells is a microscopic examination of the cells that show the degree of change from normal. How much the cells resemble the original cell is observed. Tumor cells are graded or classified as:

- **Undifferentiated cells**—These cells have an abnormal appearance and have changed greatly from the cell from which they originally developed. Usually most aggressive. High grade, grade four.

- **Poorly differentiated cells**—These cells have lost most of the characteristics of the cell from which they came. Usually aggressive. High grade, grade three.

- **Moderately differentiated cells**—These cells have changed but still resemble the parent cell. This term is used to describe cells between the well differentiated and poorly differentiated stages. Moderately aggressive. Intermediate grade, grade two.

- **Well differentiated cells**—These cells are very similar in appearance to the cell from which they evolved. Usually least aggressive. Low grade, grade one.

USC/Van Nuys Prognostic Pathologic Classification — Ductal Carcinoma In Situ

Treatment for ductal in situ carcinoma (DCIS) is undergoing change. Some physicians use the USC/Van Nuys Prognostic Pathologic Classification to determine if a patient could be a candidate for breast conservation rather than mastectomy according to various pathological studies performed on the tumor.

The grading system was developed by Dr. Mel Silverstein. In this pathologic evaluation, four categories are observed and a score is given to each category. The total score is used to determine who may qualify for various treatments. Ask if your physicians use this method of evaluation for DCIS.

1. Nuclear Grade	**Grade Value**	Evaluates size and shape of nucleus of cells
Non-high grade without necrosis	1 point	
Non-high grade with necrosis	2 points	
High grade	3 points	
2. Tumor Size	**Grade Value**	Evaluates size of the area where DCIS is found
1.5 cm and under	1 point	
1.6 cm to 4.0 cm	2 points	
4.1 cm or greater	3 points	
3. Tumor Margins	**Grade Value**	Evaluates distance from DCIS to margins of surgical specimen
1.0 cm or greater	1 point	
0.1 - 0.9 cm	2 points	
0.1 cm or under	3 points	
4. Age at Diagnosis	**Age Value**	Factors in age at diagnosis
Under 40	3 points	
40-60	2 points	
Over 60	1 point	

Final Cumulative Total
    4 points – no difference in survival-free local recurrence lumpectomy with/without radiation therapy
  5-8 points – significant decrease in local recurrence with radiation therapy
9-12 points – high rate of local recurrence, mastectomy recommended
		Total of the scores in the above four areas determines final grade

The Scarff/Bloom/Richardson Tumor and the Elston Grading Scales

Some pathologists use the Scarff/Bloom/Richardson scale or a slight modification called the "Elston Grade" for grading invasive tumors. These grading systems give a number from 1 to 3 according to aggressiveness of three different characteristics of the tumor: (1) tublar formation, (2) nuclear size/shape, and (3) cell division rate.

The numbers from each characteristic are then totaled to determine the aggressiveness of a tumor. The higher the number, the more aggressive the characteristics of the tumor.

1. Tubular Formation **Grade Value** Majority (>75%) 1 point Moderate degree (10–74%) 2 points Little or none (0-9 %) 3 points		Evaluates cell arrangement for characteristics of looking like a small tube
2. Nuclear Shape/Size **Grade Value** Uniform nuclear shapes 1 point Moderate increase in varying shapes 2 points Marked variation (often large nucleus) 3 points		Evaluates size and shape variation of cells and nucleus of cells
3. Cell Division Rate **Grade Value** Low (0–5) 1 point Moderate degree (6–10) 2 points High (>11) 3 points ***Cell Division Rate** (Elston Grading Scale Modification) **Grade Value** Low (0–9) 1 point Moderate degree (10-19) 2 points High (>20) 3 points		Determines how many cells are visible in the dividing stage in an area of the tumor * These numbers vary according to the Elston Grading Scale.
Final Cumulative Total **Points** Grade 1 – well differentiated 3–5 points Grade 2 – moderately differentiated 6–7 points Grade 3 – poorly differentiated 8–9 points		**Total of the scores in the above three areas of evaluation determines final grade**

Prognostic Tests

Various tests may be performed on your tumor by your pathologist to look at specific characteristics of the tumor cells. Tests may include:

- **Flow Cytometry**—A test that looks at the genetic material found in the DNA of a cell. Normal DNA of a cell appears with two sets of chromosomes. DNA index determines DNA composition of cells. Ploidy can be identified in the tumor, assessing potential aggressiveness. **Diploid** means having two sets of chromosomes, which is normal. **Aneuploid** refers to the characteristic of having either fewer or more than two chromosomes. This is an abnormal cell.

- **Cell Proliferation Rate**—Flow cytometry can also identify the number of cells dividing, called the S-phase fraction. This information allows a physician to know approximately how rapidly the cancer was growing (mitotic rate) at the time of surgery. A high S-phase fraction means the tumor is more aggressive. Other tests that may be ordered to measure the rate of growth are **thymidine labeling index (TLI)**, **mitotic activity index (MAI)** and **Ki67**. These tests measure cell proliferation and may also be referred to as **cell kinetics**.

- **Hormone Receptor Assay**—Hormone receptor assay is a test that measures the presence of estrogen (ER) and progesterone (PR) receptors in the tumor cell nuclei. It tells the physician whether the tumor was stimulated to grow by female hormones and is very important in determining what type of treatment will be used after surgery. If a tumor is positive, that means it was stimulated by estrogen or progesterone and usually carries a more positive prognosis.

Tumors may be:

ER positive (+) PR positive (+)

ER positive (+) PR negative (-)

ER negative (-) PR positive (+)

ER negative (-) PR negative (-)

- **Blood Vessel (Vascular)** or **Lymphatic Invasion** A microscopic examination of the tumor will show if the surrounding blood vessels or lymphatic vessels have been invaded by the tumor. No invasion offers a better prognosis.

- **HER-2/neu**—A prognostic indicator that is over-expressed or amplified in about 25 to 30 percent of breast cancers. Elevation of HER-2 indicates a more aggressive cancer. However, identification of elevation indicates that a drug called Herceptin® that targets the HER-2/neu receptor is an appropriate treatment choice.

- **p53**—Determines elevation of oncogenes (substances within cells that promote tumor development) to predict potential recurrence.

- **Tumor necrosis**—Observes the death of cancer cells inside the tumor.

There are many other diagnostic tests being used to evaluate tumors. Your physician will discuss with you the tests selected to evaluate your tumor. Each of these tests helps to collect pieces of the puzzle needed for the oncologist to determine your best treatment.

The pathologist prepares a written report that is sent to your physician. Time varies as to when the final report will be available. If the diagnosis reveals cancer, the pathologist's findings will help the physician determine which surgery and treatment will be needed. Further diagnostic tests, such as additional blood work, a bone scan, liver scan, chest x-ray, CT scan or an MRI (magnetic resonance imager), may be ordered.

When all the results are received from the tests, your cancer will be **staged** on a scale from zero (in-situ cancer) to four (a cancer with distant metastasis). A stage zero cancer is the earliest form of breast cancer and has the best prognosis. Staging is an estimate of how much the cancer has spread and is important in the selection of appropriate treatment.

The three basic factors considered in staging are (TNM): <u>T</u>umor size (T)
Lymph <u>N</u>ode involvement (N)
<u>M</u>etastasis to other areas (M)

Breast Cancer Stages 0 - 4

STAGE 0

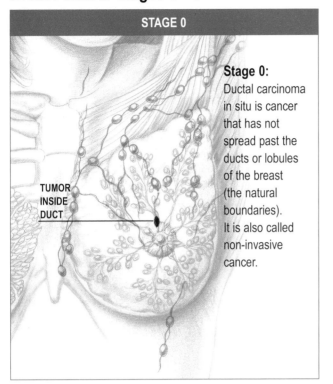

TUMOR INSIDE DUCT

Stage 0:
Ductal carcinoma in situ is cancer that has not spread past the ducts or lobules of the breast (the natural boundaries). It is also called non-invasive cancer.

STAGE I

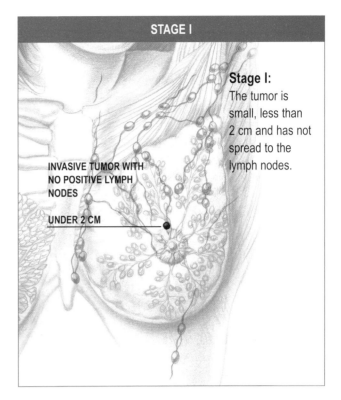

INVASIVE TUMOR WITH NO POSITIVE LYMPH NODES

UNDER 2 CM

Stage I:
The tumor is small, less than 2 cm and has not spread to the lymph nodes.

STAGE II

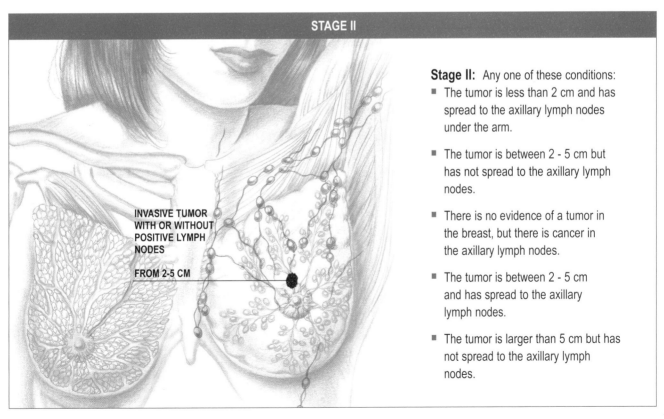

INVASIVE TUMOR WITH OR WITHOUT POSITIVE LYMPH NODES

FROM 2-5 CM

Stage II: Any one of these conditions:
- The tumor is less than 2 cm and has spread to the axillary lymph nodes under the arm.

- The tumor is between 2 - 5 cm but has not spread to the axillary lymph nodes.

- There is no evidence of a tumor in the breast, but there is cancer in the axillary lymph nodes.

- The tumor is between 2 - 5 cm and has spread to the axillary lymph nodes.

- The tumor is larger than 5 cm but has not spread to the axillary lymph nodes.

STAGE III

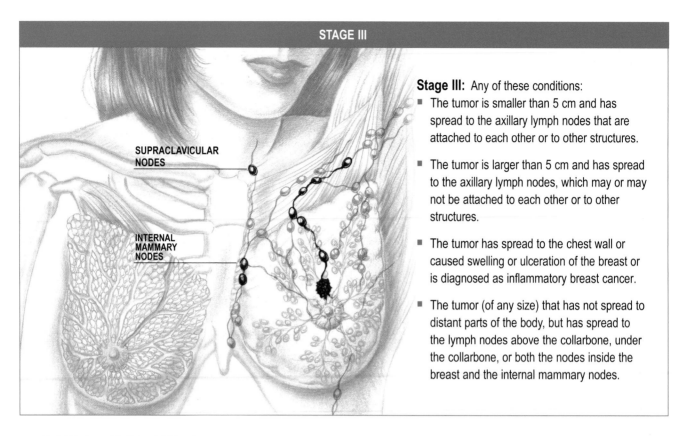

SUPRACLAVICULAR NODES

INTERNAL MAMMARY NODES

Stage III: Any of these conditions:

- The tumor is smaller than 5 cm and has spread to the axillary lymph nodes that are attached to each other or to other structures.

- The tumor is larger than 5 cm and has spread to the axillary lymph nodes, which may or may not be attached to each other or to other structures.

- The tumor has spread to the chest wall or caused swelling or ulceration of the breast or is diagnosed as inflammatory breast cancer.

- The tumor (of any size) that has not spread to distant parts of the body, but has spread to the lymph nodes above the collarbone, under the collarbone, or both the nodes inside the breast and the internal mammary nodes.

STAGE IV

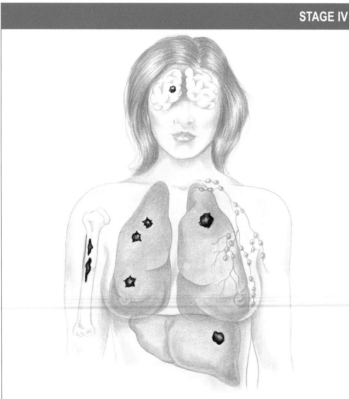

Stage IV: Distant Metastasis
The tumor can be any size and has spread to other sites in the body, usually the bones, lung, liver or brain.

NOTE:
Recurrent Breast Cancer
Breast cancer is called recurrent if the cancer has come back (recurred) after it was first diagnosed and treated. Recurrent breast cancer may occur at any stage. It may come back in the breast (called a local recurrence), in the chest wall, or in another part of the body like in distant organs, bones or other lymph nodes (also called distant metastasis), stage IV.

When you return to the physician for your pathology results, you may want to ask the following questions and write down the answers. (Some doctors will provide a copy of your pathology report for your records, and some pathologists will be happy to talk with you.) Early in your diagnostic work-up all the answers to the following questions may not yet be available.

Questions to Ask
About Your Pathology Report:

- What is the name of the type of cancer I have?

- Was my tumor in situ (inside ducts or lobules) or infiltrating (invasive-grown through the duct or lobule walls into surrounding tissues)?

- What size was my tumor? (The size is in millimeters (mm) or centimeters (cm). 10 mm equal 1 cm. 1 cm equals 3/8 inch. 1 inch equals approximately 2.5 cm.)

- Was the cancer found anywhere else in my breast tissue? The term multifocal means additional cancer was found in the same quadrant of the breast; multicentric means that it was found in another quadrant of the breast distant from the tumor. (See illustration below.)

- How many lymph nodes were removed? Sentinel node biopsy alone is usually from one to three nodes. (Approximately 75 percent of tumors have two sentinel nodes). How many levels of lymph nodes did you sample or remove? (You have three levels of nodes. Most axillary dissection removes levels one and two.)

- Were any nodes positive with cancer cells?

- Were my tumor receptors estrogen or progesterone positive or negative?

- What was my cell proliferation status? (Indicator of how fast cancer is/was growing at the time of surgery.)

- Was my tumor positive for HER-2?

- Is there anything else that I need to know about my cancer?

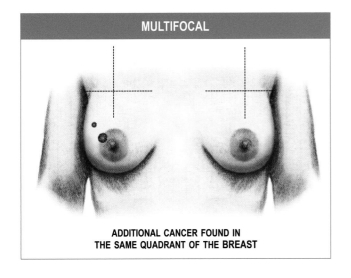

MULTIFOCAL

ADDITIONAL CANCER FOUND IN
THE SAME QUADRANT OF THE BREAST

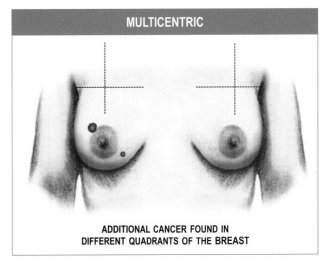

MULTICENTRIC

ADDITIONAL CANCER FOUND IN
DIFFERENT QUADRANTS OF THE BREAST

Refer to Tearout Worksheet
Tumor Location & Size - Page 203

REMEMBER

Breast cancer is a treatable disease.
It certainly is not an illness you would
choose, but it is an illness with many
proven treatments.

Acquire an understanding
of the treatment options.
This will allow you to communicate
with your healthcare team and become
an active participant in decisions.
Understanding will serve to
alleviate many irrational fears
and restore a sense of
control to your life.

Employ the best of all
medicines—your attitude.
The most productive approach
that you can bring, and one that
the physician cannot provide,
is a positive, cooperative
attitude. Determination,
combined with optimism,
creates a healing environment
that only you can provide.

UNDERSTANDING TREATMENTS FOR BREAST CANCER

"I kept a binder notebook with all my reports and labs, along with a calendar of my appointments. I asked ahead what kind of treatments they predicted would be prescribed so I could look them up. I read everything I could about the type of treatment that was being recommended. I wanted to be prepared to ask the appropriate questions before they were given. This gave me a sense of being involved in my treatment decisions."

—ANNA CLUXTON
SURVIVOR

You have had your surgery and received your final pathology report, and your cancer has been staged. The next step will be determining the need for additional treatment of your breast cancer. For a few, it will be observation only. However, the majority of women receive some type of additional treatment—radiation therapy, chemotherapy or hormonal therapy. These treatments are often called **adjuvant** (additional) **therapy**. Adjuvant therapy is given to prevent a recurrence of cancer by killing any undetected cells that may remain in your body. Adjuvant therapy may be local (radiation therapy, which targets only the area radiated to kill microscopic cancer cells) or systemic (chemotherapy or hormonal therapy, which travel throughout your body to destroy microscopic cancer cells). Your physicians will study your pathology report and tell you which treatments are indicated to be most advisable for your type and stage of cancer. They will determine which one or combination of adjuvant therapies will work best for you.

Your First Oncologist's Visit

It is very important when planning your first visit to the oncologist to carry a list of any medications that you take. Include nonprescription medicines, such as cold or sinus pills, aspirin, antacids, laxatives, vitamins and herbs, as well. Many drugs can alter the response of the treatment, and your oncologist will need to evaluate if you can continue the medication. Check with your oncologist before starting any new medication.

Your oncologist will carefully review your pathology report and any other tests, perform a thorough physical exam and then prescribe a treatment plan. This treatment plan will be designed according to:

- cancer cell type
- size of tumor
- in situ or invasive cancer
- growth rate of tumor
- evidence of cancer spreading to other parts of the body

- lymph node involvement

- how much the cells have changed from original cells

- estrogen and progesterone hormone receptor status

- HER-2 status

- your menopausal state

- your medical history

- your general health

Remember, there is more than one kind of breast cancer, and different types of cancers may require different treatments. **Do not compare your treatment with another patient's treatment** because you will probably be comparing two completely different cases. Also, the information you can get from papers, magazines, radio and television may not be applicable to your cancer. Many are reports of experimental treatments that have not been tested extensively. Rely on your physician and staff to make sure you are receiving accurate information that is relevant to your treatment.

Chemotherapy

Chemotherapy is a compound of two words that means chemical and treatment. We have all experienced treatment with chemicals for other illnesses, such as antibiotics and cold medicines. The word **chemotherapy** usually refers to treatment of cancer through the use of drugs. This is systemic treatment that travels to all parts of the body through the bloodstream. A combination of several drugs may be used to fight your cancer. The drugs selected will have different side effects and work in different ways to kill or control growth of any cancer cells at different phases of cell division that may be left in the body. Most often the drugs that cause hair loss and nausea are considered chemotherapy drugs; however, drugs that alter the hormonal environment of the body, anti-hormonal drugs, which cause few side effects, are also included in this category.

The goals of chemotherapy drugs are to:
- Destroy cancer cells in other parts of the body

- Stop cancer from spreading to other parts of the body

- Slow cancer growth

- Relieve symptoms of cancer

Hormonal Therapy

Hormonal therapy may be recommended by your oncologist. This type of additional anti-cancer therapy is prescribed after surgery for some women if their cancer pathology report revealed that tumor growth was dependent on the female hormones estrogen and progesterone. Tumors that have a significant number of estrogen receptors (ER) are considered "ER positive," and tumors that have a high number of progesterone receptors (PR) are considered "PR positive." The receptor status of the tumor determines what treatments will best affect your cancer. The use of hormonal drugs often depends upon whether you are pre-menopausal (having your monthly menstrual periods) or post-menopausal (not having your monthly menstrual periods).

Tamoxifen Citrate (Nolvadex®)

Hormonal therapy may be recommended if the studies performed on the tumor prove to be positive for stimulation by estrogen or progesterone. The most commonly used drug is tamoxifen citrate (Nolvadex®). While doctors don't know exactly how tamoxifen works, they acknowledge that it blocks the effects of estrogen on breast cancer cells. It does not kill, but it may control any remaining cancer cells that have been left in the body after surgery. It does not cause the side effects of chemotherapy. There is no hair loss or fatigue.

Tamoxifen is given by pill once or twice a day. The most frequently reported side effects from studies cited in the package insert are hot flashes (80 percent on tamoxifen and 68 percent on placebo) and vaginal discharge (55 percent on tamoxifen and 35 percent on placebo).

In studies of tamoxifen, the risks for cancer of the lining of the uterus and for blood clots in the lungs and legs increased two to three times compared to numbers recorded for the placebo group, although they occurred in only one percent of women. Women who have a history of blood clots or who require anti-coagulant medication should not take tamoxifen for risk reduction of breast cancer. Strokes and cataracts also occur more frequently with tamoxifen therapy. In addition, if you are pre-menopausal and sexually active, it will be necessary to ask the physician about appropriate non-hormonal birth control. Women who are pregnant or expect to become pregnant should not take tamoxifen. New drugs (SERMs) similar to Tamoxifen are Evista (ralosifene) and Fareston (toremifene) may be prescribed by your physician if an anti-hormonal therapy is needed.

Aromatase Inhibitors

A newer class of drugs called aromatase inhibitors, Aromasin® (exemestane), Femara® (letrozole), and Arimidex® (anastrazole), show promise in the treatment of many breast cancers in women who are naturally or are chemically made post-menopausal. The data shows that they are at least as effective as tamoxifen which has been standard hormonal treatment for breast cancer for thirty years. Aromatase inhibitors work by depriving hormone dependent cancers (ER or PR positive) by blocking or preventing estrogen in the adrenal glands. Your physician will tell you if your cancer treatment will include an aromatase inhibitor.

Biological Response Modifier

A biological response modifier is a drug that binds with certain proteins on a tumor to prevent their growth. For women whose tumors test positive for over-expression of HER2 receptors, the drug Herceptin® (trastuzumab) may be used. Herceptin® attaches to the HER2 protein found on the cancer cell to prevent it from growing or dividing. Your pathology report will show if your tumor is HER2 positive. This drug is only indicated in treatment when a tumor tests positive for over expression of HER2.

Hormonal and Biological Response Modifier Drugs

BREAST CANCER CLASS OF DRUGS	DRUG ACTION	DRUG NAMES
SERM's (Selective Estrogen-Receptor Modulators)	Drug binds to estrogen receptors in breast controlling growth	**Nolvadex**® (tamoxifen) **Evista**® (ralosifene) **Fareston**® (toremifene)
Aromastase Inhibitors	Reduces or prevents estrogen production in adrenal glands	**Aromasin**® (exemestane) **Femara**® (letrozole) **Arimidex**® (anastrazole)
Biological Response	Drug binds with certain estrogen proteins on breast cancer cells preventing growth in HER2 positive women	**Herceptin**® (trastuzumab)
Miscellaneous Hormonal	Used for breast cancers that are estrogen dependent	**Zoladex**® (goserelin acetate) **Faslodex**® (fulvestrant) **Lupron**® (leuprolide)

Chemotherapy Drugs

Chemotherapy works by killing cells that are dividing in your body, unlike the hormonal and biological response modifier drugs that prevent or slow growth. The cancer cells are constantly dividing until something disrupts this cycle—the role of chemotherapy. Even when the surgeon thinks all of your tumor has been removed, you may receive adjuvant chemotherapy because there is a possibility that some cells may have broken away from the original site and moved through the lymphatic or blood vessels to other parts of your body (metastasis) where they cannot be detected; this is called micrometastasis (the cells are too small to be detected). Adjuvant chemotherapy helps destroy these cells. Chemotherapy and hormonal therapy are effective in all parts of the body.

Because chemotherapy works by killing only dividing cells, most of the side effects will be on the cells in your body that are constantly dividing to produce new cells. These cells are found in your bone marrow, where your blood components are made, resulting in lowered blood cell counts; in the gastrointestinal tract, resulting in a possible sore throat or mouth or diarrhea; and in hair follicles, which could result in hair loss. Most of these cells are able to recover quickly when treatment is over. Therefore, these side effects are over quickly. Some people experience very few side effects and are able to continue to work throughout treatment.

Don't listen to anyone else and their stories about the side effects of chemotherapy. Instead, ask your nurse for the name of the drugs prescribed for you and the side effects of those particular drugs. There are currently about 50 drugs being used to treat cancer, and there are about 100 types of cancer, including approximately 15 different types of breast cancer. Therefore, it would be difficult to get accurate information from anyone but medical professionals involved with cancer treatment.

How Chemotherapy is Given

Chemotherapy drugs may be given by mouth, as an injection into the muscle or fatty tissues, or into a vein by an IV (intravenous) needle. Most chemotherapy for breast cancer is given intravenously. If your veins are hard to locate or you are to receive certain types of chemotherapy drugs, some doctors may request the insertion of a permanent IV device (referred to as a vascular access device, a port—"life port" or "port-a-cath"). This is a device inserted by a surgeon under the skin, usually on the chest opposite your surgery site or, occasionally, on the arm. This device may be used to draw your blood for blood studies as well as to administer chemotherapy and other medications. It prevents repeated needle sticks to your arm. You are able to bathe and swim as usual with a port.

Chemotherapy Drugs

CHEMOTHERAPY CLASS OF DRUGS	DRUG ACTION	DRUG NAMES
Anthracyclines (antibiotic-based)	Alters the structure of cellular DNA	Adriamycin® (doxorubicin) Ellence® (epirubicin) Doxil® (doxorubicin HCl liposome)
Taxanes	Prevents cancer cells from dividing	Taxol® (paclitaxel) Taxotere® (docetaxel)
Alkylating Agent	Interferes with cellular metabolism and growth	Cytoxan® (cyclophosphamide)
Antimetabolites	Interferes with cancer cell division	Methotrexate® 5-FU® (5 fluorouracil)
Miscellaneous Anti-Neoplastic	Interferes with microtubule assembly	Navelbine® (vinorelbine tartrate)

Chemotherapy may be administered in the doctor's office, a hospital or in a clinic. Most breast cancer patients take treatments in a physician's office or clinic. Some chemotherapy, however, may be administered by wearing an infusion pump (which is the size of a transistor radio and runs on batteries). An infusion pump allows continuous, around-the-clock delivery of the chemotherapy for several days at a time at home.

INTRAVENOUS PORT

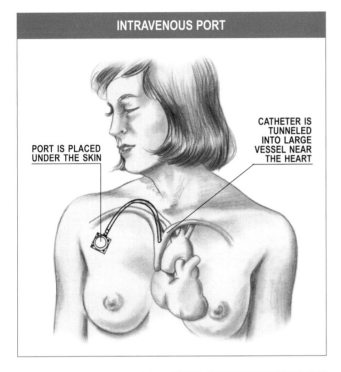

PORT IS PLACED UNDER THE SKIN

CATHETER IS TUNNELED INTO LARGE VESSEL NEAR THE HEART

PORT FILL VALVE LOCATED UNDER THE SKIN

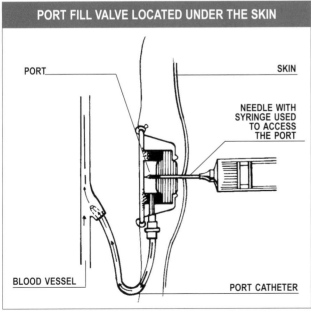

PORT

SKIN

NEEDLE WITH SYRINGE USED TO ACCESS THE PORT

BLOOD VESSEL

PORT CATHETER

Chemotherapy Scheduling

The frequency of treatments may vary, just as doses will vary from patient to patient. It will depend on the kind of cancer, the drugs being used and how your body responds to them. Some drugs are given by mouth daily. Others may be scheduled biweekly, weekly, every three weeks or by other schedules. Most breast cancer chemotherapy administered by vein is on a three or four week schedule in a physician's office or clinic. Your oncologist will be able to advise you on a treatment plan and schedule after your case has been evaluated. This schedule may be readjusted to meet your individual responses and treatment needs. Treatments usually begin after surgery; however, some types of cancer require chemotherapy administration before surgery.

Neoadjuvant Chemotherapy

Sometimes several doses of chemotherapy may be given **before** surgery to shrink a tumor, this is called **neoadjuvant chemotherapy**. Giving chemotherapy before surgery may shrink a large tumor to a size that allows for breast conservation in a woman with a smaller breast. Chemotherapy may also be given before surgery with inflammatory breast cancer or advanced stage tumors.

Dose-dense Chemotherapy

Dose-dense chemotherapy is a term used for giving the same amount (dose) of chemotherapy in a shorter period of time. Traditionally, chemotherapy for breast cancer was given on a three-week schedule, because this was the average time that it took for the blood cells to return to a near-normal level. It is now possible to shorten this period to two weeks when drugs are given to support the blood cells repopulation after chemotherapy. Neupogen® (filgrastim) or Neulasta® (pegfilgrastim) is administered to support the white blood cells return to normal range more rapidly. Red blood cells are supported with Procrit® (epoetin) or Aranesp® (darbepoetin alfa) to bring hemoglobin back up. Other drugs, Emend® (aprepitant) or Aloxi® (palonosetron), may also be given. Chemotherapy treatments can be given every two weeks if the newer drugs are used in combination with the chemotherapy drugs when needed.

Chemotherapy Side Effects

You have probably heard horrible stories about cancer treatments. Times have changed. There are new drugs that have changed many treatment side effects. Newer drugs for nausea have greatly reduced vomiting as a side effect. Drugs can now be given to elevate your immune response during treatment, preventing many of the infections traditionally experienced from extremely low white blood counts. Ask your nurse and doctor to tell you about the side effects of your treatment plan. Do not rely on well-meaning friends or family. Chemotherapy has been repeatedly successful in increasing breast cancer survival. (See Appendix B for types of drugs.)

Clinical Trials

Occasionally, as part of treatment decisions, some women may have the opportunity to participate in new treatments called clinical trials. These are new investigational studies that research the planning of highly effective treatment and prevention strategies. Thousands of research studies are currently under way in the United States. Most trials are conducted by the National Cancer Institute, major medical centers, or pharmaceutical companies. If a new treatment is determined safe and effective at the completion of the trial, the U.S. Food and Drug Administration (FDA) grants approval for their widespread commercial use by patients.

Four Phases of Clinical Trials

1. Phase I trials test new treatments to determine the acceptable dose and administration method.

2. Phase II trials study the safety and effectiveness of the drug and how if affects the human body.

3. Phase III trials require a large number of patients receive either the newer therapy or the standard therapy in order to compare beneficial survival results and quality of life during treatment. If the newer drug is found to be more effective than the standard one, the trial is stopped and all participants are eligible for the more successful treatment. If there is any evidence that the newer drug is inferior or has unusual toxic side effects, the experimental medication is discontinued.

4. Phase IV trials are conducted to further evaluate long-term safety and effectiveness of the trial drug after approval for standard use.

Clinical Trial Informed Consent

Your doctor or nurse will explain in detail the type and purpose of the trial. The patient will be given an informed consent form to read and sign. This form must include the expected benefits, the negative aspects, other treatment options, assurance that your personal records will be kept confidential, and a statement indicating that your participation is voluntary and that you may withdraw at any time.

Participating in the trial does not prevent you from getting any additional medical care you may need. If you decide to participate in the trial, you will need to contact your insurance provider to ask if it covers any charges. Be sure the researchers are aware if your plan does not cover the costs of clinical trials. Some trials are simply a comparison of two drugs or timing of administration to determine which is more effective. Your physician will explain the details of the trial.

Questions to Ask About Clinical Trials:

- What phase is the clinical trial now in?

- Who is sponsoring the study? (Needs to be approved by a reputable national group like the National Cancer Institute, a major teaching institution, or the FDA.)

- What is the purpose of this study?

- What advantage does this trial have compared to standard recommended treatment?

- How long will the clinical trial last?

- Where will treatments be given and evaluated while on the trial?

- Is the drug or combination of drugs available outside the clinical trial?

- How will the success of the treatment be evaluated? (blood tests, scans, etc.)

- How much additional time will participating in the trial require over standard treatment?

- Will there be any extra expenses or will all costs of the trial be covered?

- Will my insurance cover the cost of the trial?

- What type of follow-up will continue after the trial is completed?

Understanding Clinical Trials

If you want to know more about clinical trials, the most obvious place to start is with your oncologist. The Cancer Information Service (CIS), a program supported by the National Cancer Institute, can compile information about the latest nationwide cancer treatments for a specific type and stage of cancer. For more information on clinical trials, you can access the Physician's Data Query (PDQ) at www.cancer.gov/cancerinfo/pdq/cancerdatabase.

Patient advocacy groups such as the American Cancer Society (ACS), at 1-800-ACS-2345 or www.cancer.org, also have patient information on participating in clinical trials and other relevant information on new trials.

To Participate or Not to Participate

The decision is often not an easy one to make. This decision is very personal, and one that can only be made after you discuss the advantages and disadvantages with your physician and clinical trial nurse. When the final decision is made, you need to feel that you have chosen what is best for you. Some women prefer the "tried and true," while others feel that they are getting an even better chance by taking a newer drug or drug combination. Some feel that by their participation in clinical trials they will be helping other women in the future. Remember, no one has the right answer to the question of whether or not one should or should not participate; there is not an absolute answer. That is why it is called a "trial."

Questions to Ask Your Oncologist:

- What kind of treatment will I receive (chemotherapy, hormonal, immunotherapy)?

- On what schedule will I receive these treatments?

- How long will I receive treatments?

- How long will each treatment take?

- Where will I receive my treatments (office, clinic, hospital)?

- Will any other tests be given before or while I receive my chemotherapy?

- Can someone come with me when I receive my treaments?

- Will I feel like driving myself home after my treatment or do I need a driver?

- Will I need radiation therapy?

- Do you have written information on my cancer or treatment plans?

- Should I eat before I come for my treatments?

- Can I take vitamins or herbs if I so choose?

- What kind of protection precautions to my skin should I take during chemotherapy (exposure to sunlight)?

- What side effects will I experience from the treatments (nausea, hair loss, changes in blood cell counts, etc.)?

- Will I be given medications to treat the side effects?

- When I complete my treatments, how often will I return for checkups?

- How will you evaluate the effectiveness of the treatments?

- What are the names of the drugs?

- Are the drugs given by mouth or into a vein?

- Will I need a port (device implanted under the skin) to receive any I.V. medications or will you use a vein in my arm?

- Will I continue to have menstrual periods? If not, when will they return?

- Should I use birth control? What type do you recommend?

- Will I be able to conceive and bear a child after treatment?

- What physical changes should I report to you or to your nurse during treatment?

- Can I continue my usual work or exercise schedules, or will I need to modify them during treatments?

- Are there any precautions my family should take to limit exposure to the chemotherapy during my treatments (shared eating utensils, bathroom facilities)?

Refer to Tearout Worksheets
Personal Treatment Record - Page 211
Questions for Medical Oncologist - Page 217

As survivors, we fight adversity
with a desire to grow and learn.

We find resources to give us the skills to
handle what life has brought our way.

We put priority on learning about the
challenges rather than fleeing in panic.

We read, listen and reach out to those
who can give us understanding.

—*Judy Kneece*

Appreciating all of life, we can see
painful events as opportunities, for
those are the moments that truly stretch
us and expand us to grow and deepen
beyond who we think ourselves to be.

In what may seem the worst of times,
when we face loss, or tragedy,
we discover our heroism, our courage,
our love, our creativity, and our power.

These seemingly catastrophic
experiences are occasions to
stretch ourselves beyond
whoever we have been up to now
and to play life full-out.
These are profound challenges.

—*Judy Tatelbaum, author*
"You Don't Have to Suffer"

RADIATION THERAPY

"For seven weeks I made daily trips to the hospital for radiation therapy. There were four breast cancer patients scheduled within the same hour. We became good friends and still meet for lunch periodically. We bonded with the healthcare personnel as well, and almost hated to see 'graduation' come!"

—MARILYN REJ
SURVIVOR

Radiation therapy is most often given after breast conservation or a lumpectomy. A **radiation oncologist** is a physician who specializes in using radiation (x-ray) therapy to treat diseases. If your physician feels that radiation therapy could kill any remaining cancer cells in a local area of your body, you will be referred to a radiation oncologist for evaluation. After reviewing your pathology report, all diagnostic test findings and your surgery report, the radiation oncologist will perform a physical exam and write a prescription for the dosage of radiation and the exact area to be treated.

Understanding Radiation Therapy

Radiation therapy is delivered by a machine that produces high-energy x-rays from radioactive substances. The radiation is directed to the area in your body where pathology reports identified disease or potential for microscopic disease. The series of treatments has the ability to kill remaining cells in the treated area. This radiation is just like the radiation used in x-rays, only stronger. It is painless, and you cannot see the rays. Because radiation therapy lessens the size of the tumor mass and alleviates tumor pressure, it can also be used for cancer pain control. A lumpectomy is usually followed with radiation therapy to the breast area for five to seven weeks.

First Radiation Therapy Visit

On your first visit you will go through a process to calculate the exact area to be radiated. X-ray pictures or a CAT scan may be taken to determine precisely where to direct the rays of radiation. These areas will be marked carefully on your body to ensure that your treatment is delivered to the exact place it is needed. Ask your radiation oncologist how the area will be marked on your body and if there are any precautions you need to observe during treatments.

Receiving Radiation Therapy Treatments

When you go for radiation therapy, you will lie on your back on a table in a treatment room. You will be alone but monitored by a camera outside of the room. These treatments usually take only 10 to 15 minutes to deliver and are given as outpatient treatments on a daily basis, Monday through Friday.

Internal Breast Radiation Therapy

A new method of delivering radiation therapy is MammoSite® partial breast irradiation or limited-field radiation. During lumpectomy surgery, a small, soft, balloon is placed in the site of the removed tumor. The balloon has a thin catheter (tube) that is later used to insert a tiny radioactive source (seed) that delivers radiation therapy by a computer-controlled machine to the internal site. This area surrounding the tumor is the area that has the highest risk of recurrence. Treatments are usually given on an outpatient basis, twice a day for five days. The radiation source is present only during the treatment. Between treatments you are not radioactive. The balloon is removed when treatment is completed. Side effects to the skin are minimal. This type of radiation is for patients who meet strict criteria for the treatment. MammoSite® is now available in some centers. Your physician will inform you if it is available in your center and if you meet the patient selection criteria.

Side Effects of Treatment

Throughout the therapy, your radiation oncologist will check on the effects of the treatments. The side effects from the radiation are mild. Some experience mild fatigue, slight skin discoloration in the area (resembling a sunburn), sore throat, difficulty swallowing or a dry cough. Radiation treatments are painless during delivery and do not make you radioactive, nor do they make you a danger to your family.

Skin Care During Radiation Therapy:

- When bathing, use only mild soaps (Tone, Dove, Basis or baby soap) in the area being treated.

- Avoid scrubbing or vigorous wiping with a washcloth or towel.

- Avoid washing the marks off; if the marks should come off, inform your technologist.

- Avoid extremes of hot or cold to the skin; no heating pads, ice pack, hot-water bottles, sun lamps, tanning beds or sun bathing.

- Wear loose-fitting soft, cotton clothing over the treated area. A 100 percent cotton bra, tee shirt or camisole is recommended.

- Do not wear a tight fitting bra or a prosthesis that rubs the area. (Some women sew a lightweight prosthesis into a tee shirt or cotton camisole that does not fit closely to the body to wear during radiation treatments if radiation therapy is required after mastectomy. Cancer boutiques have cotton camisoles with temporary prostheses for sale.)

- Wait until two weeks after treatment to wear your regular bras or prosthesis. However, if you have a breakdown of the skin, you will need to wait until you are completely healed.

- Do not shave under your arm with a razor blade; use an electric razor.

- Do not use deodorant products during treatment.

- Do not use any powder, perfumes, lotions or other scented or alcohol-containing skin preparation on the treated area.

- If dryness occurs, ask your nurse or physician what types of cream or lotions are recommended. Avoid petroleum jelly since it is insoluble and hard to remove.

- If you notice blisters occurring, inform your nurse or physician.

- If the area becomes painful, report this to your nurse or physician.

- Avoid sun exposure to the treated area for 12 to 24 months after treatment.

Questions to Ask Your Radiation Oncologist:

- How many radiation treatments will I receive?

- On my first visit, how long will it take to mark the area that will be radiated during treatment?

- How do you mark the area that will be radiated?

- Can I wear a bra or my prosthesis?

- What kind of soap and bathing do you recommend during the treatments?

- Is there anything that I cannot use during my treatment (deodorant, perfume, lotions to the chest or back, etc.)?

- Do you have written information on radiation therapy for the breast area?

- What side effects are considered normal during therapy?

- What side effects, if they occur, should I report immediately?

Success Evaluation for Any Treatment

Absolute Risk Reduction or Relative Risk Reduction

When your physician talks about percentage of treatment success of a certain drug or combination of drugs, it is important that you ask if they are quoting figures that are based on **absolute risk reduction** or **relative risk reduction**.

Absolute risk reduction is the absolute number of patients that will benefit from the treatment. Example, if the risk of your cancer coming back is 4 percent and the medication recommended shows from studies that only 3 percent of the women had recurrence, this shows an absolute benefit of a 1 percent increase in benefit. (4% - 3% = 1%). One additional woman in 100 would benefit from the medication.

However, your physician may talk about **relative risk reduction** instead. Figures reported from the previous example (4% - 3% = 1%) would be stated as a 25 percent reduction in recurrence. This is a relative risk reduction. Relative risk reduction figures are derived by taking the absolute number and translating it into a percentage of increase or decrease of women who benefited from taking the drug. The 25 percent relative risk reduction from the above example was derived as follows:

$3/4 = 75\%$
$100\% - 75\% = 25\%$ relative risk reduction

Not knowing if your healthcare provider is quoting you absolute risk reduction figures or relative risk figures can be very misleading and confusing. If percentages are used, ask if these are absolute risk reduction figures or relative risk reduction figures. It is best to always know the absolute benefit from a drug or treatment in order to make an informed decision. Simply ask, "What is the actual number of women out of 100 that benefited from taking the drug/treatment?"

REMEMBER

Radiation therapy is used to destroy any cancer cells in the area that is radiated.

Radiation treatments are painless during delivery of the treatment.

Radiation therapy does not make you radioactive. You are not a danger to those you come in contact with.

Ask your healthcare provider about how to care for the radiated area.

Refer to Tearout Worksheet
Questions For Radiation Oncologist - Page 219

People suffer emotionally
because they do not know what else to do.
Reach out to other people for help—
counselors, healthcare professionals,
psychiatrists, and educators—to help
learn how to deal with your emotional
suffering and to learn to live
triumphantly in spite of a
cancer diagnosis.

Physical activity is most
difficult when we are feeling depressed,
but it is also one of the most therapeutic
things we can do to elevate our mood.
One of the best prescriptions
for depression is to physically move.
Walking, gardening, biking, swimming
or anything that get us up and
going are helpful for depression.

—*Judy Kneece*

COMPLEMENTARY THERAPIES

In the treatment of cancer, there are proven and unproven treatments. Treatments outside of the medical treatment team's established norm of recommendations are called alternative therapy (treatments in place of). Complementary therapy (treatments added to) may enhance the therapy recommended by your physician and others may interfere with treatment. Always discuss any form of treatment with your physician.

After a diagnosis of cancer, you will hear from many sources—friends, family and the media—about treatments for cancer. Some of the information will sound very appealing, especially when you are faced with choosing between treatments that have unpleasant side effects and those that do not. It is true that chemotherapy and radiation therapy have some unpleasant side effects; however, these treatments have proven results. They have been found effective in fighting your type of cancer. The treatments recommended by your physicians have many years of scientific study and clinical trials supporting their effectiveness. Many of the alternative therapies have never been the subjects of scientific studies, and their effectiveness has not been proven. Some healthcare organizations, including hospitals, cancer clinics, and physicians, however, are engaged in clinical trials to test the effectiveness of some alternative therapies. Choosing to forego conventional therapy and replace it with an alternative treatment calls for a critical, thorough, and wise investigation.

Before considering a non-traditional, unproved alternative therapy, ask the following questions:

- What and how much scientific evidence from clinical studies on humans has been published that explains the effectiveness of this treatment on my type of cancer?

- Are the testimonials from reputable health professionals or only anecdotal reports?

- Are the claims validated with clinical data such as x-rays or laboratory tests?

- Is the person promoting the therapy benefiting personally?

- Do the promoters claim that if the products fail, it is because of "lack of faith"?

- What will the treatment cost? Will insurance cover it?

- Can you continue your regular treatments and try the alternative therapy at the same time?

Complementary Therapies

Some complementary therapies are encouraged by physicians. Complementary therapies and activities may enhance your recovery. These may include meditation, relaxation, stress management, acupuncture, exercise such as yoga, and some diets and vitamin supplements which do not compromise your nutrition. Discuss with your physician the complementary therapies that will not interfere with your treatment and may be beneficial to you. Many healthcare organizations, including hospitals and cancer centers, have integrated these types of therapies in the treatment protocol in an attempt to provide a more holistic and balanced approach to treatment.

Cancer Treatment Terminology and Information Resources

Various terms associated with healthcare therapies, including medical or clinical, investigational, complementary, integrative, unproven, alternative, and quackery are often used to describe methods of diagnosing, preventing, or treating health conditions and diseases, including cancer. As a patient, it is important to understand what the terms mean, which approaches are considered safe, and where you can find accurate information about various types of treatments.

Medical Treatments

Medical or clinical treatments are those that have been clinically tested for years following a strict set of guidelines and are found to be safe and effective. The results of such studies have been published in medical journals and peer reviewed by other doctors and/or scientists in the field. The Food and Drug Administration (FDA) grants approval for the treatments or procedures to be used in mainstream medicine.

Investigational Treatments

Investigational treatments or research treatments or therapies are studied in a clinical trial. Clinical trials are research based projects that determine if a new treatment is effective and safe and, if applicable, the optimal dose for treatment. Before a drug, device, or other treatment can be widely and responsibly used to treat patients, it is studied and tested, first in a laboratory setting, usually with test tubes and then in animals. If these studies prove successful and safe, it is then tested on patients in a clinical trial. Patients are recruited to participate in a clinical trial and are monitored as to their response to the investigated therapy. A significant number of patients must participate in order to validate the results. If clinical trials prove the effectiveness of the treatment or drug, the FDA may approve it for regular use by healthcare providers. Only then does the treatment become part of the standard, recommended collection of proven methods used to treat or diagnose disease in human beings.

Integrative Therapy

Integrative therapy is a term that refers to the combination of both evidence-based or mainstream medicine and complementary therapies.

Unproven or Untested Methods

Unproven or untested therapies may refer to treatments with little basis in scientific fact, or it may also refer to treatments or tests that are currently under investigation. Adequate scientific study and evidence is not yet available to support its use.

Alternative Therapies

Alternative refers to treatments that are used in place of conventional medical therapies and may often be promoted as cures. Most often they are unproven because they have never been scientifically tested according to US standards or they may have been tested and found to be ineffective. Choosing alternative therapies instead of traditional medical treatments may cause a patient to put her health at risk.

Quackery

Quackery refers to the treatments, drugs or devices that claim to prevent, diagnose or cure diseases or health conditions, including cancer, that are known to be false or have no proven scientific evidence on which to base their claims. These methods are most often based on a few patient testimonials or so called "doctor" recommendations as evidence for its efficacy and safety. Often the treatment is claimed to be effective for multiple diseases as well as cancer. The elderly or chronically ill are often targets of quackery therapies.

After a cancer diagnosis, you deserve every opportunity to restore your health to optimal levels. Choosing appropriate treatments is the foundation for your recovery. Many people find that it is helpful to combine complementary therapies with treatment recommended by their healthcare providers but are often reluctant to share this decision with their physician. However, it is important to tell your healthcare providers about any treatments, therapies, drugs, vitamins, or herbal products you are considering. There are many therapies that you can safely use along with standard medical treatment to relieve symptoms, reduce side effects, ease pain, and to enjoy your life more. However, there are also some therapies that could interfere with traditional treatment and even cause harmful side effects. Recovery is a partnership between you and your physician. You must communicate to receive the best care possible.

Complementary Therapies

Complementary therapies refer to supportive methods that are used to complement or add to proven medical treatments. Complementary therapies may not be done to cure disease but rather to help control symptoms and improve general well-being. Examples of some types of complementary therapies that may support medical treatment are:

- nutrition
- aromatherapy
- herbal therapy
- art and music therapy
- journaling
- counseling
- psychotherapy
- spiritual practices
- prayer
- meditation
- biofeedback
- hypnotherapy
- healing energy
- massage therapy
- chiropractic therapy
- t'ai chi
- exercise
- reflexology
- yoga

Journaling

Writing in a journal is an effective way to handle the emotions that living with cancer has triggered. Journal writing empowers you to express your difficult feelings in a safe and private way. It allows you to come to terms with cancer at your own pace and in your own way. Your journal is always there to receive your thoughts and feelings. It helps make sense of live events, find meaning in them and learn the lesson they have to teach. Because journal writing forces you to look inward, it helps clarify your fears and thoughts. By writing, you will realize that your illness is only a part of you, not the whole person. It helps you put your illness in perspective.

Prepare by getting a notebook or use your computer and select a time you will journal daily.

Ideas for Journaling

1. Record your feelings, fears and what blessings you enjoyed or discovered each day.

2. Start a list of 50 ways cancer has changed your life; 50 strengths you have; 50 things you have always wanted to do; 50 ways to nurture yourself. Add to the list gradually.

3. Write down your prayers, if you are spiritual.

4. Collect inspirational sayings and poems.

Information Resources

The Internet is a helpful tool for self-education. However, it is also a tool that can be used to promote useless treatments with unproven outcomes. The following is a list of reputable sites providing information you may find helpful.

Alternative and Complementary Medicine:

- American Cancer Society: www.cancer.org

- CancerGuide by Steve Dunn: www.cancerguide.org

- National Cancer Institute: www.nci.nih.gov

- National Center for Complementary and Alternative Medicine (NCCAM): www.nccam.nih.gov

Herbal and Food Supplements:

- American Botanical Council: www.herbalgram.org

- Medical Herbalism: A Journal for the Clinical Practitioner: www.medherb.com

- US Pharmacopoeia Consumer Information (Botanicals): www.usp.org

Research on Alternative/Unproved Methods:

- National Council for Reliable Information www.ncahf.org

- Quackwatch: www.quackwatch.com

Complementary and Alternative Therapies:

- American Cancer Society's *Guide to Complementary and Alternative Cancer Methods*, Foreword by David S. Rosenthal, M.D., www.cancer.org

REMEMBER

There are proven and unproven
breast cancer treatment therapies.

Ask for data on alternative treatments
recommended to see if they have proven
human results available on
effectiveness of the therapy.

Keep your healthcare team informed
of any additional treatments
you receive.

Ask your healthcare team about
therapies that will complement your
treatment and add to the
quality of your life.

PROSTHESIS SELECTION

"The day I was fitted with my prosthesis was a major step in my road to recovery. For the first time in weeks, I began to feel that life just might return to normal again."

— HARRIETT BARRINEAU
SURVIVOR

Restoring your body image after breast surgery is an important part of recovery. A prosthesis is a form molded as a breast and is worn inside your bra. Prostheses vary from a soft fiber filling placed in your bra to a custom-made form of your breast. Some women prefer not to leave the hospital without a way to appear balanced in their body image. To make this possible, a temporary soft prosthesis, a fabric form that can be filled with fiber filling to match the size of the remaining breast, can be placed into a bra. When the incision is healed a permanent prosthesis can be selected.

Temporary Prosthesis

Ask your nurse where to find a temporary soft prosthesis. Some hospitals or the American Cancer Society's *Reach to Recovery* program provide patients with a temporary soft prosthesis.

If you desire to purchase your own temporary prosthesis, check with your local prosthesis fitter. You can find the names located in your phone book under Prosthetic Devices, or you can ask your surgeon's staff for recommendations. Prosthetic shops specialize in custom forms, and you can purchase soft, front-opening bras and a form you fill with a soft

fiber to match the size of your remaining breast. Some women have found it helpful to purchase these items before their surgery. This allows them to restore their body image soon after a mastectomy and before they can be fitted with a prosthesis.

Wearing a Bra

Women who have breast-conserving surgeries (lumpectomies) usually are more comfortable with a bra immediately after surgery to prevent movement of the remaining breast tissue. A well-fitting bra can prevent discomfort caused by excessive movement of the breast tissues. Sleeping in the bra can also be helpful.

Mastectomy patients often find that wearing a bra right after surgery is uncomfortable and tends to rub the incision area. They feel more comfortable braless while wearing a soft large, cotton sweatshirt until their incision heals. Some find a man's cotton tee shirt is a good choice and can be worn under their clothing. A cotton exercise bra, found in any department store, is comfortable for some. Others are comfortable wearing a lightweight bra with a temporary prosthesis of fiber filling. Some choose to go braless at home and wear their lightweight bra and prosthesis when going out. You be the judge of what suits your needs best, either a soft bra or braless. **However, do not wear any bra that rubs or causes irritation to your incision while it is healing**. Reconstructive surgery patients need to ask their reconstructive surgeon for recommendations on wearing a bra during the weeks following surgery.

The lightweight temporary prosthesis presents a problem—the bra rides up and causes the prosthesis to be higher on the chest wall. This can be corrected by anchoring the bra to other undergarments (panties) with a piece of elastic which is attached by snaps or Velcro, pinned or sewn on, to hold the bra down in position. Weights, such as those used in curtains and found in fabric shops, may also be sewn into the bra cup on the prosthesis side to add weight and prevent the bra from riding up.

Post-Mastectomy Bras

Special post-mastectomy bras are available, but many women prefer to purchase a prosthesis that fits in their favorite bra. This bra should **not** have **underwires** and must fit well. The fitter can help you decide if this is possible with your existing bras. She can show you how to create a pocket in which to place the prosthesis in order to prevent it from falling out. There are models that adhere to your body, allowing you to wear your own bras.

Permanent Prosthesis Selection

When your incision has healed, usually four to six weeks following surgery, your physician will give you a prescription for a prosthesis, which allows you to file for insurance coverage for the prosthesis. Do not be fitted until your surgical site has healed. For some patients this may take longer.

When ready to shop for a prosthesis, it is best to make an appointment for a fitting with a trained prosthetic specialist. The specialist will help you decide on a prosthesis according to your breast size, the weight you need in a prosthesis and your life-style. Plan to go when you have time to look carefully at all she has to offer so you can find the prosthesis that best suits your needs. A fitting usually takes between one and two hours. When you go for your fitting, take or wear a close-fitting garment so that you can see what your body looks like with the prosthesis. Some women have found a man's cotton tee shirt is easily accessible. If possible, take a friend or your mate with you, someone who can see how the prosthesis looks and who will give you an honest opinion.

Types of Permanent Prostheses

Breast forms, like our breasts, come in many shapes and sizes. They may feel rubbery and very much like your own skin. They may be covered with a soft fabric, polyurethane or a silicone envelope. Some are filled with foam rubber, chemical gels, polyethylene material, polyurethane foam or silicone gel.

Like natural breasts, prostheses vary in weight, and their consistency varies from soft and pliable to relatively firm. They are also designed for the right and left side. Some have nipples that will appear much like your remaining breast. Forms are designed to fit into special pockets inside mastectomy bras to prevent the prosthesis from falling out.

There is also a model that attaches to your skin with a sticky adhesive or a tape that is applied to the skin so that when you move, it moves. This model also prevents the riding up of the prosthesis in the bra, which is a problem for many women. If you feel this would be appropriate for your lifestyle, you may ask to try the adhesive and tape. Wear it for several days to be sure that you do not have an allergic reaction. This prosthesis can be worn with your regular bras, and you can also go braless.

If you have reconstruction and do not have the nipple reconstructed, there are nipple prostheses. Women that have had segmental mastectomies or lumpectomies may need a prosthesis called an equalizer, which is designed to fill in the section of tissue removed from the breast.

Altering Clothing for Prostheses

You can also learn from the fitter how to alter your swimsuits for use with your prosthesis. Extremely lightweight forms are available for use with your nightgown or leisure clothes. Many clothing items such as sportswear, lingerie and swimsuits that accommodate a prosthesis are also sold in prosthetic shops.

Some women buy silky, lacy camisoles and sew lightweight prostheses inside to wear under their nightclothes and when they do not want to put on their regular prosthesis.

Questions to Ask Your Prosthesis Fitter:

- How do I clean my prosthesis?

- Can I get it wet?

- How long will it take to dry?

- Does perspiration damage the prosthesis?

- Will pool chemicals cause any damage?

- Is there an exchange policy if I decide it does not meet my needs?

- How long should the prosthesis last?

- How much will my insurance provider pay toward the cost?

- Does my insurance company pay for mastectomy bras?

- If yes, how many bras will my insurance pay for at my initial purchase?

- How often will my insurance provider pay replacement costs of my prosthesis?

- How often will they pay for replacement bras?

- If I alter them, can I wear my regular bras with my selected prosthesis?

- Do you bill the provider for the cost, or do I pay and bill my provider?

What Prostheses Cost

Prices range from a few dollars for fiber filling up to around $350 for a permanent prosthesis. Most women spend around $250 for a prosthesis. Custom-made prostheses and prostheses that adhere to your body are more expensive. Bra costs start at $20 and go up.

Most professional shops will assist you in finding out what your insurance company or Medicare will pay on your prosthesis and bras. **Some insurance policies state that they will only pay for a prosthesis or reconstruction**. If you plan to have reconstruction later, this may prevent the provider from covering the cost of your surgery if you file for the cost of a prosthesis. **Check your policy or call your provider if you plan for later reconstructive surgery**.

When You Cannot Afford a Prosthesis

If you cannot afford a prosthesis, some local American Cancer Society units have loan closets. Women who have had reconstruction may donate their prostheses to be given to other women who cannot afford one. Call your local American Cancer Society to ask if they provide this service.

The Y-Me organization has a Prosthesis and Wig Bank to provide women who have financial needs with a free breast prosthesis or a wig, if they have the appropriate size of prosthesis or color of wig available. A small handling charge is requested, and the product is mailed anywhere in the United States. The telephone number is listed in the resource section at the end of this book.

Ask your healthcare team if they know of any sources that assist women in the purchase of a prosthesis after surgery. Some local organizations may offer this type of support for patients who cannot afford to purchase needed prosthetic devices.

REMEMBER

Plan to shop for a prosthesis
when you have time to carefully
evaluate which breast form best suits
your need. Make an appointment
with a specialized fitter.

Take someone with you who will be
supportive and honest in helping you
evaluate how it looks. Take a tee shirt or
tight sweater to try on over the new
form to see how it looks
under clothing.

Do not try to save a few dollars on a
prosthesis you do not like or feel
comfortable wearing. Restoring your
body image is a very important
part of recovery.

MONITORING YOUR EMOTIONAL RECOVERY

"My physical recovery went well. At first, it seemed, so was my mental and emotional state. After three or four months, things began to change. I knew people still cared, but the initial interest and concern began to wane. I was still surrounded by so much love, yet I was feeling totally alone."

—HARRIETT BARRINEAU
SURVIVOR

"My one-year diagnosis anniversary blind-sided me a little bit. My mother sent me a huge bouquet of pink roses to work and I broke down crying. But I still reflect back upon the entire thing as a gift of change. Going to a support group, even months afterwards, is incredibly helpful too. Getting involved in breast caner advocacy work has helped me with the need to give back and continue the fight."

—ANNA CLUXTON
SURVIVOR

The unexpected diagnosis of breast cancer can serve as a threat to a woman's life, self-esteem, body image, sexuality, social life and career. Many confusing emotions accompany the diagnosis as these threats are individually worked into your life; however, most women manage to cope successfully. Tears are a natural and expected response, just as occasional periods of depression are natural. This natural depression after a loss is called a **reactive depression**. Scattered throughout the months after your surgery and during treatment, you will have periods of feeling down. Reactive depression is a common emotional state after a loss and is expected after the diagnosis of breast cancer. However, it is essential to understand the difference between a normal reaction of feeling depressed and clinical depression, which requires intervention by health professionals.

Reactive Depression

In the future, sometimes for no known reason or because a situation has upset you, you may find yourself feeling blue, down, or depressed. If the feeling lasts for several days and then you begin to feel better, this is a normal reaction (reactive depression) after a major loss in your life.

It is helpful to realize that these periodic feelings of sadness, which last for several days, may occur in the future. However, these periods of depression should be short-term. These often occur on:

- **Anniversary dates:** Dates of diagnosis, surgery or treatments can cause an "anniversary reaction." These dates may bring back vivid memories and feelings experienced during these events in the past. It is normal for these dates to create a sad reminder of the experience, but anticipating and planning can significantly reduce the emotional strain.

- **Check-ups:** This same depression may occur around the time for a return visit to your physician for a check-up after breast cancer. We refer to this normal reactive depression as "check-up anxiety." Most women are anxious the week or days surrounding their check-up, wondering if anything new will be found. If the exam is negative, the blue mood lifts.

- **Treatment conclusion:** Another time many women feel depressed is at the conclusion of all their chemotherapy or radiation treatments. This depression is referred to as post-treatment depression and is very common.

It can be helpful if you anticipate these times and plan your activities to accommodate for your "blue" feelings. Plan a special time away from your routine duties to do something special, spend time with friends or arrange a light schedule of work. At the conclusion of treatment, set new goals to do things that you have always wanted to do.

For some women, incorporating this major loss into their lives becomes a problem. Their depression and tears do not cease; they continue for extended periods of time during or long after surgery and treatments are completed. These periods may occur often or remain as a constant companion. This may signal a need for additional help in making the adjustment psychologically.

Depression That Needs Intervention

It is helpful if you recognize the difference between a normal reactive depression to your diagnosis and one that signals clinical depression (depression that needs professional intervention). Clinical depression is a serious condition with real symptoms that affect both the mind and the body. Symptoms are prolonged, severe and increasingly incapacitate your ability to return to normal functioning. The positive fact is that clinical depression usually responds positively to counseling and medication. The majority of people who seek help for depression find their treatment successful.

The first step in distinguishing the difference between feeling blue and clinical depression is to know the warning signs and not feel uncomfortable about seeking appropriate help. Women can be helped to overcome depression and live a normal, healthy life. "Feeling blue" or periodic depression means that one may feel sad but can still enjoy and look forward to parts of life, such as a family gathering, a movie or seeing a friend. **Clinical depression**, on the other hand, is often manifested by:

- Continuous (week after week) feelings of sadness during or after surgery and treatment

- Social withdrawal from friends or family

- Feelings of worthlessness

- Excessive feelings of guilt

- Excessive feelings of fear of the future

- Being very slow in physical movement or speech

- Constant jitters or nervousness with no apparent reason

- Low energy level; feeling tired all the time

- Inability to make decisions

- Negative thinking, constant anger or mistrust

- Imaginary health problems

- Obsessions about health and cancer

- General disinterest in food or eating excessively

- Disinterest in work or day-to-day activities (things which used to interest you)

- Disinterest in intimacy or sex

- Insomnia (inability to sleep, waking early or being unable to go to sleep)

- Hypersomnia (sleeping too much, wanting to sleep all the time)

- Suicidal thoughts (If you have suicidal thoughts and feel that death would be an easy choice, please call your physician or nurse immediately.)

If you find that you are experiencing several of these symptoms (some experts say five) for a period of two weeks or longer during or after treatment completion, **your physician should be notified**.

Treatment for Depression

Depression may be treated in several ways. For mild cases, counseling may be all that is needed. Counseling identifies weaknesses in coping skills and works to strengthen them. Often, talking to an understanding person accomplishes much for a depressed person. Medication may be needed to assist the process. Antidepressants, medications used to treat depression, are often prescribed and generally take up to two weeks to provide positive results. A nutritious diet and regular exercise have proven to be beneficial in reducing depression and stress. A professional healthcare provider can evaluate an individual and determine the most appropriate type of help. If you are experiencing depression, know that this is **not** a sign of weakness. Many breast cancer patients have a struggle adjusting. This is a legitimate condition that is experienced by many people after a major crisis or loss. Breast cancer patients also have to deal with hormonal fluctuations caused by treatment, increasing the potential for depression. These hormonal fluctuations may cause radical changes in emotions that may necessitate intervention for relief.

After breast cancer, most depression persists for a **short** period of time, and short-term counseling or medication can help you through this period of adjustment. **Identifying and seeking help is the first step** to resolving the problem of depression. Most patients respond well to counseling or medication. **If you are experiencing depression, consult your physician**. Asking for help is a **sign of strength**, not weakness.

Medications called SSRIs (Prozac®, Zolfoft®, Paxil®, Luvox®, Celexa®) have proven effective in treatment for both depression and anxiety. They are also helpful in the treatment of hot flashes associated with menopausal symptoms during breast cancer treatment. Another antidepressant, Wellbutrin®, is available for patients who do not have anxiety with their depression. Wellbutrin® has no sexual dysfunction associated with use. Your healthcare provider will evaluate your symptoms and select the appropriate medication if needed. The good news is that most patients respond positively with intervention for depression or anxiety.

REMEMBER

Plan to keep your friends and family involved in your life while undergoing treatments. They are a great buffer against stress. Ask for help when you need it.

Depression is not a sign of weakness.

Depression is common after a major loss or crisis.

Most depression is generally short-term and usually responds to counseling and/or medication.

Seeking help for depression is a sign of strength.

Self-Evaluation for Depression

A simple self-evaluation can help you determine if you should seek help from a healthcare professional. Read the following statements and place a check mark rating the frequency you experience these symptoms or feelings ranging from never to all of the time.

Symptom	Never	Occasionally	Often	All of the Time
Feel no pleasure or joy in life				
No longer interested in things that once brought pleasure				
Avoid spending time with family or friends				
Difficult to make simple decisions				
Feel guilty				
Feel sad and blue				
Feel angry at others				
Feel mistrustful of others				
Feel trapped in circumstances				
Want to sleep all the time				
Can't sleep long without waking up				
Constantly think about my cancer and health				
Feel uptight or anxious about future				
Constantly feel tired or exhausted				
Lost or gained weight				
When good things happen, I don't feel happy				
Lost interest in sexual intimacy				
I feel helpless				
I feel hopeless				

If you find that most of your ratings fall in the category of often or all of the time, please call your healthcare provider. There are interventions that can help reduce and restore your former mood. Do not suffer in silence.

The first recommendation for depression is to start a program of walking or other form of exercise. Aerobic exercise improves mood and is good for the heart and bones as well. The next is to talk to a professional counselor. This helps identify the cause of your mood change. The final step is to add medication to enhance the process.

CHAPTER 15

SEXUALITY AFTER BREAST CANCER

"Resuming sexual relations with my husband after surgery was not easy for me. I was not comfortable with my own sexuality and wasn't sure what I wanted or expected from my husband. Fortunately, he was more comfortable with this than I was. He very tenderly and lovingly helped me come to terms with this part of our recovery."

—HARRIETT BARRINEAU
SURVIVOR

"We had to learn to navigate my new body. It was important for us to resume the intimate part of our life as it was the one thing we and we alone shared. Also, after the tremendous assault on my body, we looked upon the tenderness together as healing."

—ANNA CLUXTON
SURVIVOR

Breast cancer has changed many things in your life. One of the potential changes may be in the area of your return to normal sexual functioning. Women share that their sexual attractiveness to their partner was of primary concern during their recovery. Many factors are involved in successfully adjusting to the change breast cancer has brought. It is helpful if you evaluate your present status and take steps to restore any areas that may not have returned to normal.

A woman's breasts play an important part in her femininity, and any breast surgery or disease will threaten her sense of being a female. This is a normal response. However, it is important that you take steps to incorporate these changes into a healthy perspective that allows you to return to your former state of functioning. Changes brought about by surgery are often related to your personal view of your new body image.

Focus Group Research

EduCare Inc. conducted research during 2000 and 2001 on sexuality after breast cancer treatment in focus groups of breast cancer survivors. The groups were convened in 11 different hospitals nation wide. The purpose of the groups was to gather information from women who had taken chemotherapy and on the impact it had on their sexual functioning and quality of life. Investigated were the physical changes experienced, the sexual changes, the impact on the relationship with their sexual partner, their educational needs before treatment, and the women's request for future services of pre-treatment education and support to be offered by their healthcare team and facility.

Judy C. Kneece, RN, OCN conducted the focus groups, with patients invited by their healthcare facility. A total of 126 survivors responded to 143 questions using individual Audience Response Interactive data pads. These hand-held computer pads allowed all answers to be anonymous. Each woman was free to express her true feelings without anyone knowing how she answered. The computer automatically analyzed the data entered at each individual site and then combined the 11 sites for the final analysis.

Your Body Image

One of the hardest and most important steps is viewing the incision area and the changed or missing breast. This is indeed difficult, but it is an essential step to recovery. Your mate will share your pain and loss and, when allowed to participate in this sensitive area, will have the doors opened to respond to your needs. Not allowing your mate to participate will build a wall of separation that will affect the sexual relationship.

Breasts add pleasure to the sexual relationship but are not essential for sexual pleasure to occur. It is not the loss of a breast that changes the relationship as much as the way you and your mate accept the loss. Facing the loss together and openly communicating about how your surgery may change your sexual relationship are the first steps in successfully adjusting. The earlier this is done, the smoother the transition to recovery.

It is helpful to plan to view the surgical scar as early as possible. The first dressing change is a good choice, if possible. However, some women find that they prefer to find a time more emotionally suitable to them. The goal, however, is that you allow your sexual partner to view your new body image. This is an important step to restoring normal intimacy. Delaying may even make it more difficult.

SURGICAL SCARS

- Partners' viewing of scar: 75 percent replied that it was within days after surgery.

- Perception of partners' response when viewing the scar: 80 percent reported their partners were accepting and supportive. 15 percent reported a neutral response and 5 percent reported a negative response.

- 6 percent reported that their partner had never seen their scar. These women still dress or undress behind closed doors or in the dark.

Resuming Physical Intimacy

When can you resume intercourse after breast cancer surgery? As soon as the two of you would like. If no complications arise, the incision should heal in about four weeks following surgery. However, you may resume your sexual relationship before the area is totally healed. The best time to continue is when both of you feel ready. The surgical scar area will naturally be sore or sensitive, but you can lead your partner in how to prevent pain by altering positions to avoid pressure on the breast.

Some women have shared that even though their mates had viewed the incision, they found difficulty in participating in sexual intimacy unclothed. This problem was solved by purchasing a lacy camisole that could be worn with or without a prosthesis. Most camisoles purchased at a cancer boutique have a pocket to place a soft fiberfill or your prosthesis. For some, this helps to preserve their feelings of femininity during the sexual relationship. Examine your feelings carefully as to what may be preventing you from resuming your sexual relationship with the one you love.

Surgical Side Effects on Sexuality

During the period surrounding your diagnosis and surgery, sexual functioning may be affected by emotional stress or physical fatigue from surgery. This is a normal interruption that will be time-limited and, when over, should not impair your former state of sexuality.

It is understandable that sexual feelings are naturally diminished during high periods of stress. However, during periods of stress the need for emotional closeness increases. Most women express that they really need and want more touching, hugging, and emotional closeness during this stressful period of their diagnosis and surgery. But they often don't know how to express this need or are afraid to ask. You may also feel unsure about how to respond and find yourself withdrawing. Do not allow walls of silence and emotional isolation to separate you from your partner. This will diminish your physical closeness during this time because your partner is not sure how to treat you. Let your partner know you still desire to be close and to touch but that you do not feel up to sexual intercourse. Your partner will appreciate your honesty. They, too, are having to sort through this new emotional experience.

Radiation Therapy Impact on Sexuality

Radiation therapy to the breast area ranges from five to seven weeks of daily treatment (Monday through Friday). If the patient is not getting chemotherapy, radiation starts several weeks after breast surgery or when the incision is healed. If you are having chemotherapy, radiation usually follows the chemotherapy.

During radiation treatments, you are not radioactive and sexual contact can continue. However, you may notice that you may experience increased fatigue during treatments, resulting in diminished sexual interest. When radiation treatments are completed, you will find there is no lasting impact on the sexual relationship if you have/are not taking chemotherapy or hormonal therapy.

Chemotherapy Impact on Sexuality

Side effects from surgery and radiation are short term. If additional treatments with chemotherapy are required, sexuality changes become more of a long-term challenge because of the impact of the drugs. Most chemotherapy teaching for patients is about the well-known side effects of fatigue, nausea, vomiting, and hair loss. Very few couples are forewarned about the impact on their sexual functioning, other than the potential for infertility if the woman is pre-menopausal. The problem is that chemotherapy most often causes instant menopause in pre-menopausal women, and increases menopausal side effects for menopausal women.

Menopause caused by chemotherapy is different because it occurs suddenly, unlike normal menopause that occurs over years. The symptoms with chemically induced menopause are more intense because the drugs diminish the hormones made in the ovaries and the adrenal glands. Normal menopause causes a reduction in the ovarian hormones of estrogen, progesterone, and eventually testosterone; the adrenal glands continue to supply some hormones, causing symptoms to be less severe.

The other important factor to understand is the production of testosterone. Testosterone is predominately a male hormone, but females also make testosterone in the ovaries and convert hormones made by the adrenal gland. Testosterone is the hormone that produces sexual desire and the ability to experience an orgasm, as well as governs the intensity of the orgasm. When a woman takes chemotherapy, she has an instant reduction of all female hormones along with testosterone from both the ovaries and adrenal glands. Side effects of the reduction of estrogen and progesterone are very apparent—hot flashes, night sweats, mood changes, and vaginal dryness. However, the side effects of testosterone reduction are seldom recognized and are often ignored. Because the symptoms are experienced by the patient and impact only her and her partner, they are very rarely addressed. By understanding all of these changes, their causes, and interventions to reduce side effects, your sexual relationship with your partner should not suffer but thrive because you are actively seeking interventions to deal with side effects. We will briefly discuss the major side effects.

Fatigue

Obviously, after chemotherapy treatments your energy level will be low. You may not feel like doing much of anything for several days or weeks after each treatment because of lowered blood counts, which cause fatigue. Fatigue will vary with the type of drugs you receive. Ask your physician about the drugs and expected levels of fatigue.

Fatigue has a cumulative effect, increasing as treatment progresses. Plan to get additional rest by taking naps or sleeping in when possible. Reduce as many tasks of daily living as possible during your highest levels of fatigue. Take the initiative to divide household responsibilities among family members or even consider hiring help during this time. Most women are least fatigued the week before treatment.

This is the time to plan activities requiring more energy. You may be physically and emotionally exhausted during treatment, but this will improve.

Be sure that your meals are nutritionally adequate; good nutrition is required to build new cells to replace those that chemotherapy destroys. You may be too tired to prepare nutritionally balanced meals and may need help in this area. Treatments will end, blood counts will increase, and energy will return gradually. It is important to know that the return of energy does not happen in days or weeks when treatment is completed but that it requires months; some women even say a year passed before their normal levels of energy returned. Look at this as a time to take good care of yourself physically.

FATIGUE

Women participating in the sexuality study indicated their energy level at the time of diagnosis was 7.6
(1 = no energy, 10 = high energy).

When asked how chemotherapy impacted their energy levels:

- 62 percent reported a decrease from their baseline energy during treatments

- 40 percent reported a decrease six months after completion of treatments

- 22 percent reported a continued reduction at one year after completing treatment

---

Nausea and Vomiting

Nausea and vomiting used to be major side effects of chemotherapy, but with new drugs, they can be controlled in most cases. It is important that nausea and vomiting be controlled because they increase fatigue, decrease nutritional intake, and increase the potential for electrolyte imbalances. Report any uncontrolled nausea or vomiting to your healthcare team.

Mood Swings

When women lose their estrogen, through natural or chemical menopause, one of the first things they notice is a change in their emotions. Before menopause, this is experienced the few days before their menstrual period and referred to as premenstrual syndrome (PMS). You are probably well aware that this time is emotionally different. PMS occurs when estrogen and progesterone fall to their lowest levels to allow menstruation. During these few days, increased moodiness, tearfulness, nervousness, and outbursts of anger are common symptoms in many women. The same symptoms occur during reduction of female hormones from chemotherapy. A sad fact is that some women feel that their unstable emotions are caused because they are not "handling cancer" well or that they are depressed. The fact is, their bodies are thrown into the same emotional limbo as PMS, but it remains day after day because the hormones do not return to reverse the withdrawal. This emotional roller coaster is caused by the chemotherapy drugs and not your emotional weakness or ability to "handle cancer."

MOOD SWINGS

Participants in focus groups reported an increase in emotional mood swings:

- 55 percent increase in mood swings during treatment

- 42 percent increase six months after treatment ended

- 19 percent increase at one year after completing treatment

Mood changes after chemotherapy are an expected side effect and vary in degrees of intensity. It is almost a certainty that mood changes will occur during treatments. The reduction of the female hormones caused by treatment may cause wide fluctuations in your moods. You may swing from normal to sad, then to angry, then to depressed, all with no apparent cause.

It is important to understand that this is not from emotional weakness on your part. The emotional battle is not a choice, but a side effect of treatments.

What can a woman do about her mood swings? She can discuss the problem with her physician and ask for a medication called an SSRI (Selected Serotonin Reuptake Inhibitor), which increases the levels of serotonin that elevate mood. The brand names are Celexa®, Paxil®, Prozac®, Effexor® and Zoloft®. The great thing about these drugs is that they have also proven successful in reducing hot flashes and nervousness and decreasing insomnia.

Vaginal Dryness and Painful Intercourse

Hormonal changes cause the vagina to have less lubrication, resulting in vaginal dryness. Estrogen is the hormone that causes the wall of the vagina to be soft and pliable. With the reduction in estrogen, the vagina becomes very dry. Along with the dryness, the vagina will not lubricate adequately during sexual arousal. If this problem is not understood or corrected, these problems can result in painful intercourse, and possibly a small amount of bleeding after intercourse. Painful intercourse is not pleasant and bleeding can scare both partners. There are interventions that can help, including two types of over-the-counter interventions. One is a vaginal moisture-replenishing product in the pharmacy (Replens® or Vagisil®) designed to maintain the moisture in the vagina. Vaginal moisturizers are applied inside the vagina on a regular basis, several times a week, to restore and hold moisture. They are like a facial moisturizer applied to keep moisture in. They are not designed as a lubricant before intercourse.

The other over-the-counter intervention is a vaginal lubricant. This is applied prior to intercourse to increase lubrication. Astroglide® is highly recommended by patients as being the most like natural lubrication. Vaseline® can promote vaginal infections and should not be used as a lubricant for intercourse. You should generously apply the lubricant in the vagina and on the outside on the vaginal lips. It can also be applied to the partner to increase lubrication. It is important that the lubricant be reapplied as needed during intercourse.

It is very important for a support partner to know that this vaginal dryness is not from lack of desire from the patient, but from the inability of the walls of the vagina to lubricate caused by the chemical menopause. Often, partners take this reduction of vaginal lubrication as a lack of desire for them as a sexual partner and feel rejected. Some partners feel that the use of lubricant is a sign that they are not sexually stimulating to their partner. Neither is true. Lack of vaginal lubrication is caused by chemical menopause. This is something you, the patient, cannot control.

Vaginal dryness is not only uncomfortable; it can also cause itching from dryness. The dryness of the vaginal tissues can also set up an environment for irritating or painful vaginal infections that interfere with sexual pleasure. Any itching or swelling should be reported to the healthcare team for a vaginal infection evaluation. Infections may be caused by an overgrowth of bacteria that causes a thin, gray discharge that has a fishy odor. A fungus (Candida albicans) normally found in the body can experience an overgrowth (often caused by antibiotics) causing a discharge that has a thick, white (cottage cheese like) clumps that cause itching accompanied with internal and external swelling. Both of these vaginal infections can easily be treated with medications. If you experience any vaginal discharge that is irritating or has a foul odor, report this to your healthcare provider.

VAGINAL DRYNESS
Vaginal dryness from chemotherapy was reported to increase: ▪ 123 percent during treatment   ▪ 134 percent six months after treatment ended   ▪ 160 percent one year after completion of treatments

---

PAINFUL INTERCOURSE FROM VAGINAL DRYNESS

Painful intercourse increased:

- 137 percent six months after treatment

- 149 percent one year after treatment completion

These figures reveal that vaginal dryness with the potential to cause painful intercourse increases **after** treatment is completed. Therefore, couples should be prepared to deal with the lingering side effects.

Vaginal Dryness Options

During natural menopause, women are offered oral or transdermal (patch applied to skin) hormone replacement therapy to relieve their symptoms. During breast cancer treatment, at this time, this is usually not an option. However, after treatment is completed, if the vaginal dryness continues even though vaginal moisturizers and lubricants are used, discuss other options with your healthcare provider. The first option would be estrogen vaginal cream applied inside the vagina and on the external vaginal lips. Another option is a vaginal ring of estradiol (Estring®) that is inserted into the vagina and remains in place for three months, slowly releasing the drug before replacement is needed. These localized estrogens relieve vaginal dryness and decrease urinary symptoms. After several months the vagina increases in moisture and elasticity, making intercourse far more comfortable. However, only you and your healthcare provider can determine if either option is appropriate for you.

Urinary Problems

When estrogen levels are reduced, urinary symptoms are a common side effect. Estrogen receptors are found in the lining of the urinary bladder and tubes. When estrogen levels are low, the lining becomes thinner and some women experience burning during urination, urinary urgency, and urinary stress incontinence (loss of urine when walking fast, running, or sneezing). They find holding their urine difficult and

often a source of embarrassment. The use of estrogen vaginal cream or Estring® will also greatly reduce these symptoms.

Orgasm Ability

After treatment with chemotherapy the ability to experience an orgasm during intercourse is reduced for most women. However, a small percentage of women will not suffer this side effect. Hormonal reduction usually continues to create problems for those women who remain in a permanent menopausal state. It can cause an inability to experience an orgasm or reduce the intensity of orgasm if one is experienced. Sexual arousal is also a challenge. One woman in the focus group described her sexual desire after chemotherapy as "that of an 11 year old girl." Diminished sexual interest, sexual thoughts, sexual arousal, and orgasm are all common side effects of chemotherapy.

SEXUAL INTEREST

Sexual thoughts prior to diagnosis:

- 88 percent of women reported having sexual thoughts and fantasies before chemotherapy

- 32 percent had sexual thoughts and fantasies during treatments

- 41 percent reported sexual thoughts and fantasies one year after treatment completion

When questioned about the need for extra time to achieve sexual arousal:

- 86 percent replied that the time for sexual arousal required had increased

- 49 percent reported decreased nipple sensitivity from sexual arousal

- 80 percent reported lack of vaginal lubrication

Orgasm Ability Before and After Chemotherapy

ORGASM	NEVER	RARELY	OCCASIONALLY	MOST OF THE TIME	ALL OF THE TIME
Before Treatment	1%	8%	19%	55%	17%
During Treatment	24%	27%	28%	16%	5%
One Year After Treatment	10%	23%	29%	30%	9%

Before treatment, 72 percent of women would experience orgasms, varying from most to all of the time. During treatment this fell to 21 percent. Following completion of treatment, this number rose only slightly to 39 percent, translating into a 54 percent reduction in ability to experience orgasms most or all of the time, one year after treatment.

It is important to understand that the loss of testosterone—the hormone that causes interest, arousal and orgasm is the basic problem. What can be done about these side effects? The testosterone can be brought back into normal range by a trained, experienced healthcare provider who understands the complexity of hormonal balance. Many healthcare providers are completely unaware of this intervention. Some contend that they don't know if it is safe. However, those women who have had their levels brought back into therapeutic range with local creams applied to the vaginal area report that this brought back the quality of sexual life they enjoyed before treatment. Ask your healthcare team if they check hormonal levels or supplement testosterone. If not, contact the International Academy of Compounding Pharmacists (800-927-4227) and ask for the nearest compounding pharmacy. Your local pharmacy can refer you to the providers in your area who are skilled at testing levels of existing testosterone, and prescribing testosterone cream to be applied to the vaginal area to bring levels back to normal.

Wellbutrin®, an anti-depressant, has proven helpful in increasing libido and the ability to have an orgasm for some women. Some women also report weight loss. If you have a history of anxiety or other disorders, the medication may not be appropriate. Ask your healthcare provider if you are a candidate for this medication.

Return of libido and ability to have an orgasm is a quality of life issue. It has nothing to do with life and death issues and for this reason may be ignored. For some couples, return of libido is important to their quality of life. Yet, for others, this is not an issue of importance. Only the two of you can decide what is best for your relationship. There are no right or wrong answers, only what best meets your needs as a couple. It you find that this is an important issue, keep seeking a healthcare provider that addresses your problems, offers interventions, and works to improve your quality of life.

Partner's Understanding

It is essential that your sexual partner understand the potential changes that chemotherapy may bring to your sexual functioning. One of the major differences is your increased time for sexual arousal. After chemotherapy there is a need for increased foreplay. Understanding this helps both of you approach the sexual relationship with a clear understanding of problems and potential solutions.

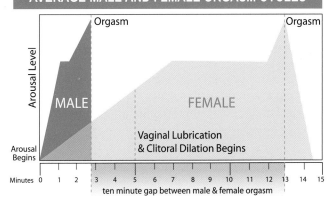

AVERAGE MALE AND FEMALE ORGASM CYCLES

The majority of women interviewed (89 percent) said they would like to have their healthcare provider explain changes in sexuality occurring from treatment to their partner. If you feel this would be helpful to you, ask your healthcare provider to include your partner in the discussion of potential sexual changes from chemotherapy.

Talking to Your Physician

Some women feel that their physicians are only interested in saving their lives and not in their daily life functions. This is NOT true. Physicians are well aware that quality of life is one of the main components of a successful recovery. Because they do not ask about sexuality problems does not mean that they will not discuss and help you with any of your concerns. Don't hesitate to ask questions and report any side effects.

Breast cancer has not changed you. You may experience some new problems after your surgery and treatment for cancer that may challenge you and your mate; but you are still the same loving person your mate selected, and breast cancer does not change that fact. Many couples share that the experience of cancer brought them closer together, and the meaning of the sexual relationship was enhanced because of the realization of how valuable they were to each other.

Restoring Sexual Function Self-Evaluation:

- Have I allowed my mate to see my scar? Am I still hiding in the closet to change clothes?

- Have I talked openly about my fear that our relationship will change?

- Have I expressed my desire for our sexual functioning not to be affected because of my cancer diagnosis?

- Have I shared openly about what is physically comfortable or uncomfortable during intimacy since my surgery?

- Am I honest when I am physically fatigued and would like to be held and cuddled without intercourse?

- Does my partner understand the potential side effects from chemotherapy on sexual functioning?

- Have I explained to my partner that when I do not feel up to the sexual act, I either need time to adjust or it is from fatigue caused by treatment, I am not rejecting them?

- Have I planned a special time and saved energy for the sexual relationship to be resumed?

- Have I been honest and asked for family assistance with household duties during treatments to allow me more time and energy for pleasurable events?

- When I have problems, such as hot flashes, dry vagina, painful intercourse or lack of sexual desire due to treatment side effects, do I talk with my healthcare team about how to manage the problems?

- Have I had my body image restored with a well-fitted prosthesis or had/or planned for reconstruction?

- If interested in reconstructive surgery, have I talked to a physician and received the information needed to make a decision?

- If I am having problems adjusting to my body image or sexuality, have I asked to speak to a counselor?

- Have I asked my treatment team or called the American Cancer Society for information on sexuality after cancer?

- Have I treated myself to a feminine treat to enhance my feeling of femininity after surgery such as a lacy camisole, perfume, an item of clothing, or a new haircut?

Readjustment in the area of sexual functioning is a common occurrence in breast cancer patients. There are many things you can do. There is help you can receive to assist the return to your normal sexual role. Don't allow changes to occur without reaching out to your healthcare provider to ask for information and, if needed, referral to professionals in the area of sexual counseling. The earlier you address these problems, the easier they are to solve. Educational material is available, and trained counselors can help you with the transition.

Birth Control After Breast Cancer

It is necessary to discuss with your healthcare provider what type of birth control to use after your surgery. Chemotherapy usually stops your menstrual periods, and they may or may not return after the treatments are completed. If you are near menopause, they may never come back. However, if you are young, they may return. For some women, several years may go by before normal menstruation begins again. Because you may be fertile (able to conceive a child) before evidence of a menstrual period, you may want to discuss with your physician the type of birth control that is suitable for you. **Do not take any oral contraceptives** (birth control pills) **without talking to your oncologist**. Alternate methods of birth control may be recommended according to the type of treatment you receive.

Note on Tamoxifen

The anti-estrogen drug, tamoxifen (Nolvadex®), may increase ovulation (release of the egg from the ovary) when therapy is started. After receiving tamoxifen, women may be more fertile. **Some method of birth control is recommended**. Discuss with your physician what types of contraception are most suitable and the length of time recommended to prevent pregnancy.

REMEMBER

The key to preventing changes in the sexual relationship is open, honest communication with your mate and your healthcare team.

Viewing the incision site as early as possible removes the greatest obstacle to restoring the relationship.

Surgery and radiation therapy may cause temporary interruption in sexual functioning due to stress and fatigue. This interruption is temporary.

Chemotherapy may cause chemical menopause in many women impacting sexual desire, sexual arousal, ability to experience orgasm along with vaginal dryness causing painful intercourse.

Your sexual partner needs to understand that these side effects are from treatment and not your lack of desire for them as a partner.

Seek help from your healthcare team for any physical problems you experience.

Ask about the need for contraception.

You are still the same loving person your mate selected. Breast cancer does not change that fact.

Survivors learn that their sexuality is a complex issue. It is more than alteration or loss of a breast; it is how we feel about our total self after cancer. We have to remember that cancer does not define who we are. We are still the same loving person who has gone through an experience that can change us into a more sensitive and caring person.

Sexuality issues are quality of life issues; they are not life and death issues. Only you and your partner are aware of the particular problems. Survivors know that quality of life issues are individual and that getting help, whatever it may be, to restore your quality of life is essential.

Survivors know that taking care of their personal appearance increases sexual self-esteem. Do what you need to —lose weight, start an exercise program, get a new hair cut, purchase some new clothes. However, always be mindful that the most sexually attractive part of you is your attitude. Positive, loving attitudes are the greatest sexual attraction. If you are emotionally stuck, reach out to a professional counselor for help. You deserve it and so does your sexual partner!

—*Judy Kneece*

THE SINGLE WOMAN AND FUTURE INTIMACY

If you are single or divorced, a cancer diagnosis can add additional stress by impacting your view of future emotional, physical and sexual intimacy. Like many other patients, you may find it difficult to comprehend how you would handle a future intimate relationship. Some women reported in our sexuality focus groups that after their cancer diagnosis and treatment, they felt as if they were "damaged goods" and that they would not be sexually attractive as a partner. This is not true! Many women have successfully managed to develop intimate relationships after a diagnosis of breast cancer.

Single women often need help understanding the impact of diagnosis on developing future relationships. The first thing necessary is for you to rethink the subject. Cancer does not define who you are. You are still the same you! Most often a cancer diagnosis causes a person to become a stronger and more sensitive person. This life experience makes you a more attractive person. Unlike some diseases, breast cancer is a treatable disease, and after treatment most women return to a normal state of physical and emotional health.

The first step is to make peace with yourself and take the steps needed to rebuild your self image, whether it be reconstruction, getting into physical shape or developing new skills. This is an opportunity for you to decide how you would like to change or improve.

When thinking about dating in the future, remind yourself:

- Dating was not always successful before your diagnosis.

- Dating after cancer will be same; sometimes it is just not the right person and has nothing to do with your cancer diagnosis.

- Most people deal with personal "defects." Some are overweight, bald or are not physically "Mr. America."

- One third of Americans will have a cancer diagnosis. Ask yourself, if this person had a history of testicular or prostate cancer, would you reject them?

One of the best ways to prepare for a future relationship is to talk to other breast cancer patients about their experiences in developing intimacy after their diagnosis. Support groups are a great place to talk to other women. The Young Survivors Coalition listed in the reference section of this book is another excellent resource. Professional counselors are also an excellent place to have your fears and concerns addressed and to make plans for how to deal with them in the future.

You need to prepare how you will share your diagnosis when you do find a new partner. Understanding how other women have handled the issue will give you a sense of preparedness and allow you to develop your own plan.

Sharing Your Diagnosis

Sharing the details of your diagnosis with a new partner should not occur on the first date. The best time is when the relationship has passed the mutual friendship stage and is progressing. However, you should share before the relationship becomes serious or intimacy may occur. Only you know when this is happening. When you feel the time is right, select a time and place where you will feel comfortable discussing your diagnosis. If you should become upset, you need to be in a place where you would not feel embarrassed.

Tips for Sharing the Details:

- State that you desire respect and honesty in your relationship and you have something you need to share.

- Share the facts about your diagnosis honestly and openly.
  "In (year) I was diagnosed with breast cancer. This required that I have a (mastectomy/lumpectomy) that was followed by (type of treatments). I have been cancer free for (time) or at the present I am dealing with (problems). I feel that what I went through has allowed me to become a stronger person by having to deal with a lot of hard issues. I wanted to be very honest with you before this relationship progressed. I will be happy to answer any questions you have about my diagnosis, treatment or present health."

- Do not appear as a victim; you do not want pity!

- Ask your friend what they think about what you just told them.

- Allow them to talk.

Remember, if this person leaves the relationship after this, this is a person that would have deserted you in the future if things did not go well. You did yourself a favor and prevented future heartaches. The nature of relationships is that some work and some don't. Your goal is to protect yourself emotionally by sharing early enough to find out if this will impact the relationship before you fall in love.

As a single woman you need to be prepared to deal with discussing your diagnosis with future partners with confidence. Surround yourself with understanding peers as you work through the process of preparing what you will say in the future. Cancer has not "damaged" you; it has been a tool for expanding your ability to love and appreciate life.

REMEMBER

Being diagnosed with cancer does not change who you are.

A cancer diagnosis can serve to make a person stronger and more sensitive.

You are not "damaged goods." You are a person who has expanded their ability to love and appreciate life.

FUTURE FERTILITY

"We were newlyweds when I was diagnosed. This raised a lot of questions about our future for becoming parents. Would chemotherapy rob us of the anticipated joy of one day having our own children?"

—ANNA CLUXTON
SURVIVOR

One of the issues least thought about during a cancer diagnosis is the impact of cancer treatments from chemotherapy and hormonal therapy on future fertility. Most thoughts naturally focus on the patient and getting the most appropriate treatment for control of the cancer. However, one of the most important issues for younger couples who have not started or completed having their family is taking the time to discuss the potential impact on their future fertility. These questions are essential for couples to ask to protect their fertility or plan for future alternative fertility methods.

For women, infertility is the inability to start or maintain a pregnancy. Infertility can occur because of the inability of the ovaries to produce mature eggs (oocytes) for ovulation. It can also occur from the inability of the body to successfully allow implantation of a fertilized egg into the uterine wall or to maintain growth after implantation.

Women and the Fertility Cycle

When a woman is born, she has all of the eggs (approximately 200,000 immature eggs) she will ever have and does not produce more. When the female hormones gear up at puberty she experiences the development of secondary sex characteristics such as breasts, pubic hair, and menstruation. Eventually, the menstrual cycles are accompanied by the release of a mature egg at mid-cycle (ovulation, around day 14) ready for fertilization by the male sperm. If conception does not occur, or if the fertilized egg does not successfully implant into the uterine wall, the prepared ovarian wall sloughs off, evidenced by the menstrual flow. The entire process begins again for another monthly cycle. Each full cycle averages from 28 to 32 days.

Each ovulation reduces the number of stored eggs. It is estimated that approximately 500 eggs reach maturity and are released over the fertile period of a woman's life. Eventually, as hormonal levels decrease, the supply of eggs that mature is reduced, ovulation ceases, hormones decrease to pre-menstrual levels, and eventually the menstrual periods stop. This cessation of ovarian function with the loss of fertility is called menopause. With menopause comes symptoms of not only infertility, but also hot flashes, vaginal dryness, changes in moods, urinary changes and others.

Fertility Threatened by Chemotherapy Treatments

Surgery has no effect on fertility, other than creating stress that causes changes in the hormonal balance that may temporarily alter ovulation and possibly menstruation. This usually resolves itself in several months. Radiation therapy to the breast alone has only temporary effects, similar to surgery, because of stress and fatigue temporarily altering hormonal functioning. The major cause of infertility, however, comes from chemotherapy.

Chemotherapy drugs work to treat cancer by killing rapidly dividing cells throughout the body. Chemotherapy drugs are cytotoxic (cyto=cell, toxic=poison). These drugs kill cancer cells, but in the process kill healthy, rapidly dividing cells as well. Shortly after chemotherapy administration, women notice hormonal changes in their body. The large majority of women suffer irregular or complete cessation of periods during treatment. Factors that determine the extent of their side effects and also impact their future infertility are based on the patient's age, the type of drug, or the drug combinations that may create a compounding effect of toxicity on the body. It is very difficult for an oncologist to accurately predict who will suffer side effects with their hormonal functioning. Some women have their fertility return after the drugs are discontinued, but for others, infertility may be permanent.

Factors that help predict future fertility

1. The nearer a patient is to menopause, the less likely she is to have hormonal function (menstruation and ovulation) return. The younger the woman, the more likely hormonal functioning is to return.

2. A class of drugs, called alkylating agents, has a more destructive effect on hormonal functioning. The most common one used in breast cancer treatment is cyclophosphamide (Cytoxan®). Other drugs that increase infertility in this category are melphalan (Alkeran®), and busulfan (Myleran®). Cisplatin (Platinol®) is usually considered an alkylating agent even though it works differently than the others in this category and also impacts fertility.

Addressing Issues of Fertility

Since physicians cannot predict with absolute certainty whose fertility will be permanently affected, there are steps to take to preserve your future ability to have children.

1. The most essential step is telling your healthcare team **before** treatments that having children in the future is top priority in making treatment decisions.

2. Ask your healthcare team to discuss treatment recommendations and their potential for causing infertility.

3. Ask for written information on the subject of chemotherapy and fertility.

4. Ask for a referral to a specialist in the area of fertility if you still have questions or concerns.

5. Ask for treatment protocols to be used that reduce potential for infertility.

6. Explore alternative fertility preservation options.

Alternative Fertility Preservation Options

Embryo Freezing

Hormones (like tamoxifen, proven safe to use in breast cancer patients) are used to stimulate egg production. Mature eggs are removed by a physician in a minor surgical procedure, fertilized in vitro (in a glass test tube) with sperm, frozen for future use and then stored. This procedure is called in-vitro fertilization (IVF). Pregnancy rates average 10 to 25 percent with each frozen embryo.

Egg (Oocyte) Freezing

Hormones (like tamoxifen) are used to stimulate egg production. Mature eggs are retrieved by the physician, frozen for future use and then stored (not fertilized). This method is new and at present has an estimated three percent pregnancy success rate.

Research in Progress:
Ovarian Retrieval and Transplantation

Ovaries are surgically removed by laparoscope (small incision through abdomen), divided into small strips, frozen and later transplanted back into the body when fertility is desired. Drugs are given to stimulate ovulation. Some researchers call the process ovarian grafting. This method is experimental but appears to have potential for women who will have chemotherapy that will damage her ovaries. The first successful birth after chemotherapy with ovarian retrieval and transplantation has recently occurred. Check with your healthcare team on the continued progress of research.

The procedures for fertility preservation are expensive and usually require several months for egg retrieval, which may delay treatments. At this time, most of the cost is not covered by insurance. During treatment decisions, this adds another difficult choice for some couples that still desire to have a family of their own. But this is an important consideration if future fertility is desired. It is important to know that some cancers require immediate attention.

One of these is inflammatory carcinoma, a cancer that is already systemic because of involvement of the lymphatic system and requires that treatment start within days of diagnosis. Discuss with your physician if any type of delay would reduce your chances for survival.

Optional Parenthood Choices

Some couples find that their priority during the diagnostic period is optimal cancer treatment, and that preserving fertility is not the prominent issue at this time. There are other methods that are still optional:

- Using donor eggs, if fertility does not return

- Using a surrogate mother

- Adoption

Facts about Pregnancy after Breast Cancer:

- Pregnancy does not reduce patient survival or trigger recurrence.

- Women who have had systemic chemotherapy have been able to conceive and deliver healthy, normal children with the chance of birth defects near that of the normal untreated population.

- Developing eggs exposed to chemotherapy may suffer genetic damage. Some physicians suggest a wait of six months before pregnancy is attempted after regular menstrual periods return. However, the time recommendation varies according to many other variables and will need to be given by your own healthcare team.

Questions to Ask if Chemotherapy is a Treatment Option:

- What is the predicted impact of the drugs on fertility?

- What percentage of women who take these drugs experience permanent infertility?

- Are there drugs with less potential for infertility that can be used?

- What options do I have to preserve my fertility?

- Do you make referrals to physicians specializing in fertility preservation, if we desire?

- If we decide to pursue embryo freezing as an option, will the time required to collect the eggs impact my survival outcomes by delaying treatment for several months?

- If my fertility returns, how long do you suggest we wait before becoming pregnant?

REMEMBER

Future fertility is an issue that may
not be discussed by your healthcare
team unless you bring up the subject.

If future fertility is important to you,
ask for information and referrals
to a fertility specialist to discuss options
best suited for you and your partner.

CARE OF THE SURGICAL ARM

"I give a great deal of credit to my Reach to Recovery visitor for my physical recovery. She provided me with a wealth of information. For the first time, I had something I could read and re-read. I was discovering fast the necessity of education in this new and strange world."

—HARRIETT BARRINEAU
SURVIVOR

After surgery for breast cancer, there are areas of your health that you will need to monitor. You need to exercise your surgical arm to regain your range of motion, and you need to learn how to prevent or treat lymphedema should it ever occur. Breast self-exam on the remaining breast(s) and the incision site, along with mammograms and clinical exams by a physician, will help you monitor for any potential recurrence. Dietary habits and physical exercise may help your recovery and add to your physical well-being. These are areas you can take responsibility for monitoring.

Changes in the Surgical Arm

After your surgery, sensation in the area of your incision will be diminished, and your arm may feel numb or tingly. The area under the arm (if the lymph nodes are removed) contains nerves that, if injured or cut, can cause different types of sensations. The most common are numbness and a tingling sensation. The area under your arm and the back of your arm is where the numbness usually occurs. If the nerve is stretched or injured during surgery, these sensations may improve in a few months. If the nerve is cut, the numbness will be permanent; however, this will not affect the use of your arm.

The surgical arm will feel very tight when you attempt to stretch it up over your head. Removing your lymph nodes also required the removal of an area of fat around the lymph nodes. This causes the area to feel pulled and tight after surgery, but it is temporary and will improve as you begin your exercise program and gradually stretch this area.

After surgery, your surgical arm needs to be exercised to restore your normal range of motion. (The "surgical arm" is the arm on the side of your surgery, and the "non-surgical arm" is the opposite arm.) **However, do not begin any exercises until your surgeon gives you permission**. Most physicians prefer that all drains, sutures or staples be removed before attempting an exercise routine. Ask your physician when to begin range of motion exercises. Additional instructions as to types of exercises may be provided by your physician.

Your Arm Exercise Program

When you begin the exercise program, you will find that you may tire easily and that there will be some discomfort as you attempt to perform the movements. However, you should continue to perform them to the point of slight discomfort **but not until it becomes painful**. It may take several weeks before you are able to complete some of the exercises. Work at your own pace. Your progress will be gradual. Some women find that by taking their pain medication, aspirin, Advil® or Tylenol® an hour before starting, or by taking a warm shower just prior to beginning the exercises, the routine is less uncomfortable.

Exercises should be performed on a regular basis—**preferably two or more sessions a day, 10 to 15 minutes each session**. Persistence is the key to regaining complete range of motion. Do the exercises slowly and hold the position when you get to the end of the range. This helps stretch and strengthen the muscles. Some exercises require a small rubber ball to squeeze and a broom handle or yardstick to hold in your hand. Many of the exercises may be performed either standing or sitting down.

SURGICAL ARM LIFTS

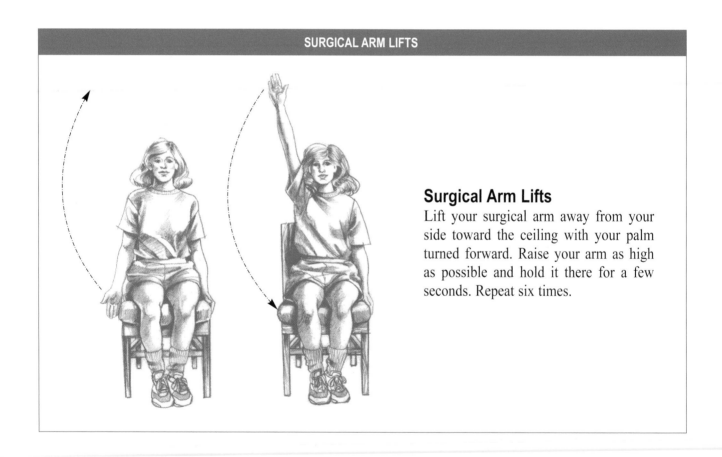

Surgical Arm Lifts

Lift your surgical arm away from your side toward the ceiling with your palm turned forward. Raise your arm as high as possible and hold it there for a few seconds. Repeat six times.

SURGICAL ARM RAISES

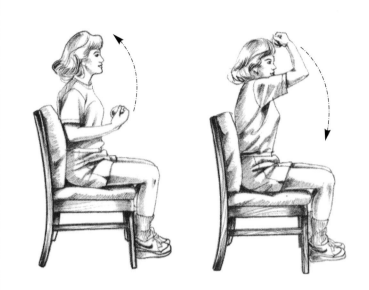

Surgical Arm Raises

Clench a rubber ball in your surgical hand with your elbow bent. Slowly lift your arm toward your head, keeping your elbow away from your body. Hold this position for a few seconds when you reach your head. Repeat six times.

SURGICAL ARM REACH

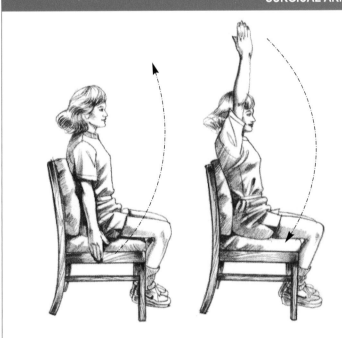

Surgical Arm Reach

Hold your surgical arm straight beside your body. Slowly raise your arm as high as possible over your head while keeping your elbow straight. Hold the position for a few seconds. Repeat six times.

SURGICAL ARM SWINGS

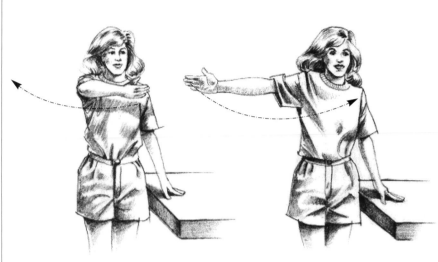

Surgical Arm Swings

Place your non-surgical arm on a table to support your body. Put your surgical arm across your chest, placing your hand on the opposite shoulder. Move the surgical arm slowly away from your body until it is extended straight out. Keep your arm at shoulder level as you perform the exercise. Repeat six times.

LATERAL RANGE OF MOTION

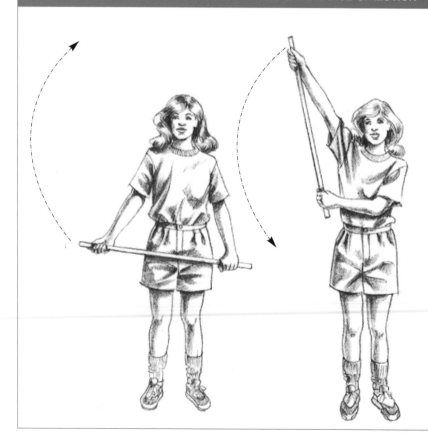

Lateral Range of Motion

Hold a stick with your surgical hand palm up and your non-surgical arm palm down, as you push your surgical arm directly out from your side toward the ceiling until you feel a stretch. Hold this position for several seconds. Repeat six times.

SURGICAL ARM CIRCLES AND ARM SWINGS

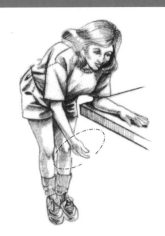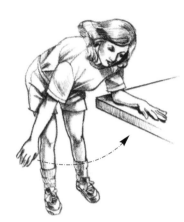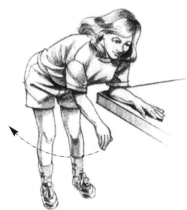

Surgical Arm Circles and Arm Swings

Lean on a table with your non-surgical arm. Move your surgical arm in a circle clockwise and then counter-clockwise. Repeat six times. Leaning on the table, as before, swing your surgical arm from side to side six times.

OVERHEAD RANGE OF MOTION

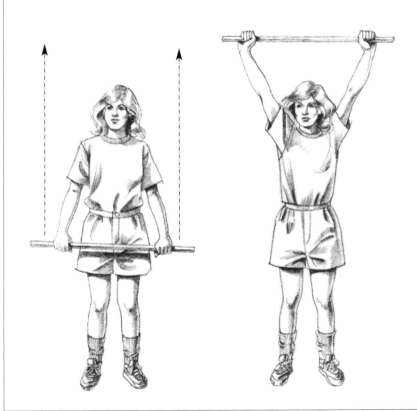

Overhead Range of Motion

Without bending your elbows, bring the stick directly over your head, leading with the non-surgical arm. Reach back over your head until you feel a stretch. Hold the position for a few seconds and repeat six times.

If you are having difficulty performing the exercises and feel you are not making progress, tell your surgeon. Some women need the assistance of a physical therapist to regain complete range of motion, or they may need the motivation of an exercise group led by a professional.

After breast surgery, it is not uncommon for some women to favor the use of their non-surgical arm and become "one armed" as they resume their daily activities. Weakness in the surgical arm, which most women experience to some degree, will cause this to happen. However, it is helpful if you remember that using the surgical arm normally will gradually increase strength and range of motion.

Lymphedema Prevention and Management

Removal of the lymph nodes under your surgical arm or radiation therapy to the underarm area may cause a swelling called **lymphedema**. (Lymph, from lymphatic fluid; edema, swelling from fluid accumulation.) Having only sentinel nodes removed will greatly reduce this potential. However, radiation therapy may cause fibrosis in some women, increasing the potential for lymphedema.

Lymphatic fluid is high in proteins. These proteins leak from vessels into surrounding tissues when vessels are obstructed. The protein then draws water into the tissues. This condition results in swelling from the slower flow and removal of lymph fluid and accumulation of protein and water in the tissues of your arm. Only a small percentage of women experience lymphedema after surgery, but all women need to know of the potential and treatment if it should occur. It can occur anytime, from shortly after surgery to years later. It is suggested that you measure or have someone measure your arm three inches above the elbow prior to surgery so you can monitor with more accuracy if you have any swelling.

Arm lymphedema can produce pain, restricted movement of the shoulder and arm, and increased susceptibility to infection. Medications and treatments are often limited in their effectiveness; therefore, the best strategy is to **prevent** the problem before it occurs.

Lymphedema may be related to:
- Surgical removal of lymph nodes
- Poor range of motion in your surgical arm
- Infection
- Obesity
- Radiation therapy to the breast and underarm area
- Constriction caused by clothing or jewelry
- Long periods of positioning the arm below the level of the heart
- Repetitious tasks using the surgical arm

The first line of defense against lymphedema is regaining the full range of motion of your arm by using the exercises suggested in this book or by your physician. While these exercises may seem dull and unnecessary, they serve to facilitate the flow of the lymphatic fluid from the arm area. **Do not begin an exercise program until your physician gives you permission**.

Steps to Help Prevent Arm Lymphedema:
- For several weeks after surgery, when lying down, prop your arm up on a pillow above the level of your heart to help drain the fluid. Elevation of the arm helps reduce swelling and prevents additional accumulation of fluid.

- Keep your arm slightly away from your body, so as not to compress the underarm area. Using a small pillow or a small stuffed animal under your arm when sitting will keep the arm away from the body and keep swelling at a minimum. Some swelling under the arm is expected due to surgery and will improve with time.

- Avoid using your arm and hand in a dependent position (below the level of the heart) for long periods of time. If you need to perform a task of this sort, periodically hold your arms above your head to promote drainage.

- Make a fist or squeeze a small rubber ball in your hand repetitively for two to three minutes several times a day to assist the accumulated fluid in returning to general circulation.

Steps to Avoid Injury and Infection:

- Do not allow the surgical arm to be used for blood pressure checks, blood samples or injections. Ask your nurse for a pink wristband or ribbon to be placed on the wrist of your surgical arm as a reminder to all your healthcare givers.

- Do not wear anything that is tight on the surgical arm or hand, such as rings, watches, bracelets or tight elastic in sleeves.

- Do not hold a cigarette in this hand.

- Do not cut your cuticles; keep hands soft by using hand lotion regularly. Avoid nail salons that use rotary files that could injure your cuticles.

- Do not carry heavy packages or purses on the side of your surgery.

- Wear protective gloves when working in the garden, washing dishes or using any irritating chemicals, such as hair dye or cleaning products.

- Avoid burns and cuts when cooking.

- Wash all cuts or injuries with antibacterial soap, apply an antibiotic medication, and cover the area with sterile gauze or a Band-Aid® until the wound heals.

- Avoid sunburn. Wear long sleeves or sunscreen at all times when in direct sunlight for a period of time.

- Use a thimble when sewing.

- Avoid insect bites by wearing insect repellent.

- Be careful with animals. Avoid scratches.

- Use an electric razor under your arm.

When to Notify Your Physician

These precautions may help you to avoid injury and potential for infection in your arm. If you ever experience any redness, pain, infection or low-grade fever after an injury, contact your healthcare provider. When accumulated lymph fluid becomes infected with bacteria and inflames the surrounding tissue, it is a condition called **cellulitis**. Antibiotics will be necessary to treat the infection. Early intervention is necessary to prevent the spread of infection to other parts of your body. If you have any evidence of redness or inflammation in your arm, your healthcare provider needs to be notified as soon as possible. This is one problem that needs immediate attention. If it occurs outside of office hours, call or page your healthcare provider.

Treatments for Lymphedema

If you have persistent swelling several weeks after your surgery, the first treatment is simply to elevate the arm. Raising the arm above the level of the heart by propping it on a pillow for 45 minutes several times a day will usually reduce most lymphedema. Sleeping with the arm elevated on a pillow is helpful. If the swelling persists after elevation, notify your physician.

Elastic Sleeve for Lymphedema

A special elastic sleeve, designed to reduce swelling, may be ordered by the physician. The sleeve looks much like support hose and can be worn under long-sleeved clothing. A professional fitter will measure the arm and make a customized sleeve to fit your measurements.

Suggestions for buying, wearing and maintaining an elastic sleeve:

- Get your physician to write a prescription for insurance reimbursement.

- Purchase two sleeves so that you can wash one while wearing the other one.

- Wash in lukewarm water and allow sleeve to air dry thoroughly. Do not wring out while wet. Do not put it in the dryer.

- Do not wear a sleeve that does not fit well. This causes skin irritation, or can increase your swelling after wearing.

- If you have a problem with the top of the sleeve rolling down on the arm, ask for a water-soluble adhesive lotion to apply under the top of the sleeve. This adhesive washes off easily with soap and water when the sleeve is removed.

- Have the fitter re-measure your arm periodically to see if the sleeve is still the appropriate size. To be effective in reducing swelling, sleeves must fit properly.

- Replace the sleeve about every six months because they stretch and lose their elasticity from repeated use.

- It is suggested that you purchase and wear an elastic sleeve on long airline flights. Pressure changes can cause an increase in lymphedema.

Lymphedema Massage

A special hand massage method, **Manual Lymph Drainage (MLD)**, also known as complex decongestive physiotherapy, is performed to remove swelling from the arm by some trained physical therapists and massage therapists. This method stimulates the skin and underlying lymphatic vessels by hand and is different from traditional massage therapy. Traditional massage may increase, rather than decrease, swelling because it is so vigorous. MLD therapists are trained to delicately move their hands over the surface of the skin slowly in circular or pumping motions to move fluid toward the shoulder. These sessions last approximately an hour or more. At the conclusion of the hand massage, the arm is wrapped in a special bandage to prevent re-accumulation of fluid in the arm. Instructions are given on how to massage the arm with the bandage in place. This method of massage and bandaging is performed several times a week for several weeks or until swelling has been reduced to a manageable level. Patients and family members are often instructed in the massage and bandaging techniques so that treatment may be continued at home.

When seeking treatment for lymphedema, always ask if the therapist is trained in or has certification in manual lymph drainage for breast cancer. If your physician does not have a recommended therapist, you can find a list of specialists on the National Lymphedema Network Web site, www.lymphnet.org.

Compression Pumps for Lymphedema

Your physician may order a sleeve hooked to a compression pump. This is a special sleeve connected to an air pump that compresses your arm. A compression pump requires several hours of time a day to manually remove the accumulated fluid. There are two types of compression pumps. One is a gradient pressure pump that has the air pressure greatest at the area of the hand with less pressure at the top of the sleeve. Another type is a sequential pressure pump that exerts pressure that starts at the hand and gradually moves up the arm to the shoulder in a milking-like fashion. Pumps are expensive and their progress is often not monitored by a trained therapist, but rather by a salesperson for the company. It is recommended that you use a pump only with a physician's order and that a trained professional monitors your progress throughout use of the pump. Overuse or too much pressure may increase swelling.

Diuretics for Lymphedema

Medications called diuretics that remove excess water from your entire body are not generally recommended for treating lymphedema. Swelling is caused by leakage of protein from the vessels in the arm. Diuretics cannot remove the protein that has seeped out into the arm. It may remove some of the water temporarily, but once you stop taking the diuretic, swelling returns because the excess protein in the arm pulls the fluid back.

Remember, lymphedema usually has **nothing to do with cancer**. This condition occurs because lymph nodes and vessels in the breast have been removed during surgery, scar tissue has formed after surgery, or radiation therapy has caused changes in the area. These conditions slow down the removal of the lymphatic fluid that accumulates in the breast and arm area, resulting in swelling of the arm and hand.

Assessing Range of Motion

After having performed your exercises for several months following your surgery, ask these questions to determine whether you have regained adequate range of motion in your arm.

If you could perform the following prior to surgery, can you now easily:

- Brush and comb your hair?

- Pull a tee shirt or sweater over your head?

- Close a back-fastening bra?

- Completely zip up a dress that has a long back zipper?

- Wash the upper part of your back in the shoulder blade area of the opposite side of surgery?

- Reach over your head into a cabinet to remove an object?

- Make a double bed?

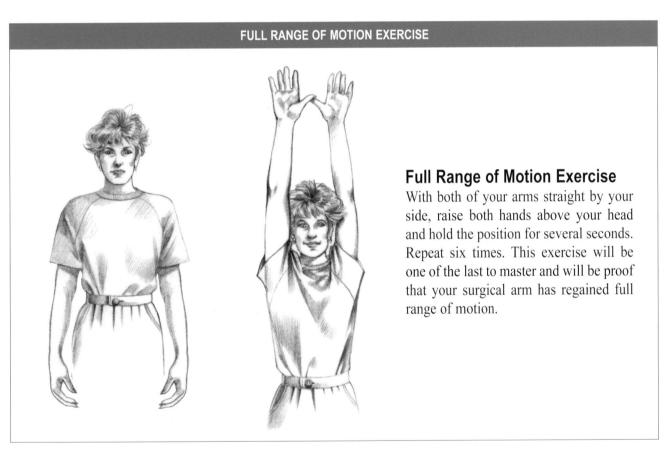

FULL RANGE OF MOTION EXERCISE

Full Range of Motion Exercise

With both of your arms straight by your side, raise both hands above your head and hold the position for several seconds. Repeat six times. This exercise will be one of the last to master and will be proof that your surgical arm has regained full range of motion.

When you can master this exercise, congratulate yourself on the hard work required to stick with your dull, routine exercise program to accomplish this task. If you have not regained your range of motion, talk with your surgeon about a physical therapist or an exercise program led by a professional trained in range of motion exercises.

REMEMBER

Exercise is essential to restore
normal use of your surgical arm.

Exercise to the point of some
discomfort but not pain.

Protect your surgical arm
from injury.

Treat lymphedema by elevating
your surgical arm. If this is not
successful, call your physician.

The best treatment for lymphedema
is prevention of swelling.

Immediately report any sign of
infection in your surgical arm.

HEALTH INSURANCE AND EMPLOYMENT ISSUES

"Nothing prepared me for the magnitude of the responsibility I would have in seeing to it that I received the insurance benefits to which I was entitled. I was overwhelmed by the number of bills I received following surgery. Good record keeping was essential."

—HARRIETT BARRINEAU
SURVIVOR

"So much to do—so little time. I made the effort to write down the name, time and date, every time I spoke with someone regarding my benefits. Don't take no for an answer. Keep everything!"

—ANNA CLUXTON
SURVIVOR

When you are diagnosed with breast cancer, inform your insurance provider and ask for guidelines for filing or payment of claims. The following questions may need to be clarified. Some of the answers may be found in your insurance policy manuals.

- Is there a need for second opinions for procedures?

- Do I need pre-approval for hospital admissions?

- How do I file claims?

- What is the name of a person at the company who can answer questions about my case?

- What is the amount of the deductible, if any, required before claims are paid?

- Are there any limits imposed on the amount paid for surgery, chemotherapy, radiation therapy or reconstruction?

- What is the policy regarding coverage for new treatments or treatments considered "experimental" (new medications or treatments)? Are there limits on what amounts will be paid?

- What is the policy regarding coverage for a permanent prosthesis? If delayed reconstruction is considered, will it pay for both, or does one exclude payment for the other?

- What is the policy for reconstruction? Does this cover surgical repair on the other breast?

Record Keeping for Reimbursement

After breast cancer, it is very important that you take steps to receive payment for services covered under your insurance. Many women find this task overwhelming. Often, a mate or a friend will volunteer to perform this job for you. Ask for assistance in this area. Keeping accurate records will make the task much easier.

Taking the Hassle out of Record Keeping:

- Keep calendar records of all appointments (a pocket calendar is helpful).

- Write on the calendar the physician you visited, procedures performed and medications purchased.

- Provide physicians with appropriate information and forms for filing claims.

- Ask for copies of **all** charges at the time of service or ask to have copies mailed to you.

- Keep copies of all charges from appointments or services **in one place** (a box, a notebook or file folder).

- Periodically check to see if payment is appropriately made to medical providers.

- If problems arise, ask your healthcare facility or provider to help you understand or assist you in providing information for adequate repayment.

- Call your insurance providers and talk with a claims representative. Offer additional records or assistance for getting information from your medical providers.

- Keep all premiums current; **do not allow your insurance to lapse**.

Insurance After Diagnosis

After any major illness, insurance is more difficult to obtain. For this reason, keep all premium payments current. If you decide to change jobs, be sure that you will be covered under the new employer's insurance program before making a decision. If you have private insurance or coverage through your employment, be very alert to these areas before making major decisions.

Financial Assistance

If your illness is going to be a financial burden to you, ask to speak to the social worker in the cancer treatment center. Social workers are trained to help you with the social issues of your illness, including helping you secure financial help for needed medical services. There are various services available, but you will need to apply for them. The earlier you can make this need known, the more effective the social work team can be in helping you file the forms. People often feel embarrassed to ask for help and postpone the issue. Many people find an unexpected illness drains their financial reserves. You are not alone. Ask for help early.

Employment Issues During Treatment

Breast cancer surgery and treatment will require some time away from your job. Most employers are very understanding and offer their support during this time. You will need to give notice of your absence and expected time away from your job.

Occasionally, however, a breast cancer patient will be discriminated against because of illness. If you have reasons to believe that your employer has treated you unfairly because of your illness, there are laws that protect you. There are federal laws and varying state laws that offer protection against discrimination or unfair practices. Listed in the reference section of this book are names and telephone numbers you can call to receive information on how to best manage your situation.

What Do You Tell Your Friends?

It is necessary for you to decide how much to tell your employer, fellow employees and friends about the details of your illness. Some women are very open about their illness and treatments. Others feel that this is a private matter and would rather not share the details with everyone. Decide what you wish for others to know. It is helpful if you inform your support partner or family members so that your wishes can be carried out when people call or drop by.

You do not have to constantly share your "illness story" with others if this makes you uncomfortable. A simple reply of "I appreciate your concern, but right now I am not up to talking about it. Thank you for understanding," allows you the right not to tell. You need to communicate, but you do not need to feel that you have to talk with everyone who asks about your illness. It may be helpful to allow family members to answer the phone and screen your calls if you would rather not talk. Plan to do what best suits your particular personality.

When Friends Don't Call or Come

Often women find that their friends don't call or come to see them after their diagnosis. This can add to the emotional pain of a diagnosis of cancer. Why does this happen?

- They don't know what to say.

- They don't know what to do.

- It hurts them to see you in emotional pain and they can't do anything about it.

- It hurts them to see you in physical pain.

- Your diagnosis serves as a reminder that they, too, could be diagnosed with cancer. It becomes easier for them to avoid you than to face their own vulnerabilities.

Breaking the Silence:

- Call your friends. Let them know that you are handling your diagnosis as well as you can and that you miss them.

- When they ask if they can help, be specific: Pick up the children, take me to lunch, pick up a prescription, drive me to the doctor, etc. They want to know that they will not add to your burdens, but can truly help you during this time.

- Invite them over for a cup of coffee or tea.

- Ask them to go for a walk.

- Be sure that you have not sent out unspoken messages that you want your illness to be a private affair.

REMEMBER

Simple record keeping will help take the hassle out of insurance filing.

Recruit someone to help with record keeping.

Keep your insurance premiums current.

Do not change jobs unless you know you will be covered by the new insurance.

If you experience discrimination on the job, seek assistance from professionals.

Decide how your friends can best help you during this time.

Don't be afraid to reach out to your friends.

SURVIVORSHIP

Worry is taking our past negative
experiences and projecting them
into the future.
This becomes self-torture and
does not prevent anything we
worry about from happening.
We have to say "no"
to our negative, defeating thoughts
or we will spend our time
in a mental prison
built from our own thoughts.

As survivors, we refuse to carry
along old resentments, grievances,
axes to grind or to remember
injustices. We know that
harbored memories grow increasingly
heavy and slow our journey to recovery.
Instead, we decide not to waste our lives
by permanently losing ourselves in sorrow,
defeat, anger, fear or guilt. We lighten
our recovery load by unloading
these energy drainers.

—*Judy Kneece*

MONITORING YOUR HEALTH AFTER BREAST CANCER

During the first year after your treatment, you will see your oncologist three or four times. If no problems arise, you will then progress to office visits several times a year. It is very important that you keep these visits with your doctor, even when you are feeling great. Other physicians involved in your care may require return visits for their area of specialty. Some women are referred back to their primary care provider.

Your physician will monitor your general health and order routine exams and screening tests to detect any recurrence or new problem. Regular blood work will be performed, and physical exams of the surgical area will take place on each visit. Bone scans, chest x-rays and other staging exams vary according to the schedule on which physicians repeat the exams. Ask about your physician's schedule for follow-up tests. Continue to have a yearly pap smear and mammograms on a regular basis. You need to ask the following questions about your follow-up care:

- How often will I need to return for a checkup?

- Do I call and make the appointment, or does your office call me?

- What symptoms should I be aware of that might indicate a possible recurrence?

- What long-lasting side effects of my treatment can I expect as normal?

- What should my arm and breast area look and feel like (painful, numb, tingling)?

- What changes might occur that I should consider dangerous and worthy of alerting you?

- Are there any special things that I should do or not do or that I should avoid (particular activities, medications, food)?

Communicating with Your Healthcare Team

Some women report that one of their most difficult tasks during treatment is communicating with their healthcare team or physician. This is a challenge, because for most, cancer is a new experience. There are so many questions, so many unfamiliar terms and so many different physicians that it is an overwhelming task to sort it all out.

Keep these things in mind:

- Know that you deserve to understand and have your questions answered by your healthcare team. This is not unreasonable; it is an important part of your recovery.

- Do not be embarrassed to ask any question. There are no silly or stupid questions, and there are many other people who have asked those same questions. Ask if you do not know.

- Realize that physicians and other members of the healthcare team are on a working schedule that allows a certain amount of time for each patient. If they appear rushed, it is not that they do not care or want to take the time; in today's healthcare economy they have to see a certain number of patients to maintain the financial viability of a medical practice.

- Understand that calling and asking to speak to a physician at the time of the call is difficult because of other scheduled patients. For questions and non-emergency situations, call and give the question to an assistant or nurse and ask to have someone call you with the answer. This may be a trained educator or physician's assistant. If you have a series of questions, call and schedule an appointment just for questions.

- Prepare to communicate effectively with your healthcare providers by reading about your disease and learning some of the new terms involved, or have a family member do this and go with you to the appointments.

- Make the most of your allotted appointment time. Forget the small talk and be sure that you are using your time to get the information you need.

- In the tearout worksheets at the back are questions that are specific to the type of physician you will be visiting. Reviewing these before the visit will prepare you to ask questions that are in the area of the physician's expertise. One physician is not able to specifically answer all questions.

- When going to an appointment with your health-care provider, it is essential to prepare what you need to tell or ask your provider in order for your physical and mental recovery to progress as smoothly as possible. Often, patients think they will remember what to report or ask during the appointment, but they leave with important questions unanswered. As you are well aware, appointment times are short and many things have to be checked by your provider. It is normal for the healthcare provider to concentrate on your physical disease and treatment. However, questions you have about quality of life side effects deserve to be brought to their attention as well. Part of being an active participant in your healthcare is being prepared to relay your physical and psychological concerns during this time in the most effective manner possible.

- If you do not understand a term or instructions, say so. Ask that they repeat or explain again. Simply say, "I'm sorry, but I am having trouble understanding what you just said, would you please explain it again?"

- Ask if they have written information on the subjects discussed.

Preparation for Your Next Appointment

Keep a written list of questions that arise between visits to ask during the appointment. If the list is long, it may be helpful to inform the nurse or give her the list of questions prior to seeing the physician. Ask if you need to make a return visit to have your questions answered.

Keep a written list of symptoms experienced between visits. Be sure to report **early** in the visit any of the following:

- Bleeding from anywhere in the body: when, amount and how it was stopped

- Fever: date experienced and temperature elevation

- Dizziness or fainting: dates

- Painful or frequent urination

- Chest or arm pain: description, intensity and date of pain

- Vision changes: type and date of change

- Constipation: frequency

- Diarrhea: frequency, including number of loose stools in a 24-hour period and number of days

- Vomiting: when, frequency and number of episodes during a 24-hour period

- Swelling in any body part

- New pain in any part of the body

- Changes in scar or breast during self-exam

Quality of Life Issues

Other areas that you should bring to a healthcare provider's attention are in the area of quality of life. Simply, these are issues that impact your ability to enjoy day-to-day activities; they are not life threatening, but they are important just the same and need to be presented in quantified terms.

- **Physical energy:** report level in understandable terms, like "unable to stay up over three hours without rest" or "unable to work."

- **Depression or feeling blue most of the time:** "I feel too depressed to participate in everyday activities with my family." "I find myself crying frequently."

- **Anxiety or nervousness:** "I feel anxious and shaky most of the day and this interferes with my ability to concentrate and interact with my family. Can you help me with this?"

- **Pain:** report on a scale from 1 (no pain) to 10 (severe pain): "I am having pain in my (area) that averages a (number you give your pain) most of the day, and this interferes with my ability to rest and participate in daily activities. Can you help me find a way to reduce my pain to a manageable level?"

- **Nausea:** report any nausea or vomiting between checkups by telling your healthcare team when and how long you were nauseated or how often you vomited.

- **Appetite:** report a reduced appetite or inability to eat.

- **Sleep:** Report inability to go to sleep or stay asleep and how long you are able to sleep uninterrupted. "I have problems going to sleep and sleep only (amount in hours) before I awake. I then find it difficult to return to sleep." "I wake up the next morning exhausted and feel sleepy during the day; can you help me with this problem?"

- **Hot flashes or night sweats:** report the approximate number you are having daily and if they awaken you at night. "I am having at least (number) hot flashes a day and they awake me at least (number of times) at night. Can you help me with this problem?"

- **Dry vagina or painful intercourse:** "I am having problems with vaginal dryness that is causing painful intercourse. Can you help me with this problem?"

- **Information needs:** keep a written list of information or referrals needed.

At the conclusion of the appointment ask when you will need to return, if there are any suspected changes that are normal that may occur before your next visit, and any changes in recommendations for your care.

As a patient you can maximize your checkup time with your healthcare providers by being prepared with your own information and by reporting anything new that has occurred since the last visit. Remember, this needs to be done early in the appointment to allow the physician time to consider if any action is needed. This makes you an active partner in your healthcare. This is the patient that every physician dreams of having—one who comes prepared to report physical status and needs, is educated on the basics of her cancer, and understands their time constraints in a medical practice.

REMEMBER

Recovery is a partnership between you and your healthcare team.

Take an active role in preparing for your appointment.

Strangely enough, I had always
looked at my body as "me."
I was unhappy when extra
pounds arrived or I got up
with a zit on my face
or I had a bad haircut.

But cancer taught me
that I am not just my body.
My body may have cancer,
but inside of this altered
physical shell is the real "me."

I am not really my body,
but I am the laughter of my spirit,
the tears of my heart, the caring of my soul,
and the loving, encouraging words
I speak—this is the real "me."

The real "me" can do things
that my body cannot do.
The "me" that resides in my body
is what people love to be with—
somehow they don't judge me on
my body, but the "me"
that resides within.

Enough said about what
others think of my body image.

—*Survivor*

DIET AND EXERCISE

"As soon as possible, I got out of the house to get into the fresh air and sunshine. I asked how soon I could start doing arm exercises and then I did them everyday. I was training to get back into life."

—ANNA CLUXTON
SURVIVOR

If your physician does not recommend a special diet, you may wish to consider making dietary changes that have proven beneficial in preventing many different health problems for other patients. Your hospital or clinic may have a nutritionist who can assist you in this process. Your goal should be to eat a balanced diet that promotes maintaining your ideal body weight while not making you feel hungry or deprived. Any diet that causes extreme hunger or is psychologically depressing is not healthy nor is it recommended for you. Avoid fad diets for weight reduction or maintenance.

Weight Gain During Treatment

Weight gain experienced by some women during treatment for breast cancer has been linked to water retention from medications, taste changes from chemotherapy, relief from nausea achieved by keeping food in the stomach and an increase in eating patterns as a result of stress. Identifying the cause of any weight gain is helpful in addressing the problem.

Diet and Health

When we talk of diet, most people think of losing weight. Almost every woman has gone on a diet to lose weight at some point in her life. However, what we eat not only affects our weight, but, of even greater importance, it also has a direct effect on our general health. Diet plays a major part in our health status and energy. As you are recovering from breast cancer, evaluate your eating habits and consider dietary changes as a healthy lifestyle choice for maximum health and energy.

Dietary fat has been linked to many diseases and is often the culprit for much unwanted weight and some illnesses. In the past, sugar has received the blame when fat was more of a common denominator. Therefore, a smart diet is monitoring what you eat to have a healthier life, and, in the meantime, you may lose unwanted pounds.

The Role of Dietary Fat:

- Dietary fat has the ability to increase the level of the hormone estrogen, which has been proven to stimulate some tumors.

- Dietary fat has been linked to higher cholesterol, which can lead to cardiovascular disease.

- Dietary fat has more calories than other types of nutrients (proteins and carbohydrates).

It is wise to lower anything that may promote disease and increase weight. For this reason, learn to count fat grams. Then learn to substitute healthy fats, mono and polyunsaturated fats, such as safflower, sunflower and olive oils, in place of saturated fats, such as animal, coconut and palm oils, which cause an elevated cholesterol level.

Learn to:

- Read labels for percentages of fat content and fat grams per serving

- Read labels for the kinds of fat

- Select foods with healthy fats

- Limit the number of fat grams eaten daily

How to Find Your Daily Allowance of Fat

Authorities recommend that women eat no more than 25 percent of their daily calories from fat. To determine how many fat grams you can eat, divide the number of calories you consume a day by four (25 percent) or by five (20 percent) to determine how many calories from fat you are allowed per day, and then divide that number by nine to convert the calories to fat grams.

Example:
(2,000 calories per day) ÷ 4 = 500 calories per day from fat

(500 calories from fat) ÷ 9 = 55 grams of fat per day

AGE	WEIGHT	FAT BUDGET
25 - 50	110-130 lbs.	65 grams
	130-150 lbs.	75 grams
	150-170 lbs.	85 grams
51 & older	110-130 lbs.	55 grams
	130-150 lbs.	65 grams
	150-170 lbs.	75 grams

Counting Fat Grams

If you wish to lose weight, you may reduce your number of grams to a lower number but do not go on a totally fat free diet. This is not healthy. Between 15 and 25 percent of daily calories should come from dietary fat. Dietary fat contains essential daily nutrients.

Now that you have determined the number of fat grams you can eat per day, find a fat gram chart and select the foods you may eat on a balanced diet that does not leave you feeling hungry or deprived.

Tips to Help You Maintain a Low-Fat Diet:

- Eat more chicken, turkey and fish instead of red meat (remove skin; do not fry)

- Broil or bake meat; cook with nonstick skillet and use cooking spray

- Buy fat-free or low-fat salad dressings and mayonnaise

- Buy low-fat cheese

- Try frozen yogurt for dessert instead of ice cream

- Look at fat grams in bread (most are low-fat, but a croissant is high in fat)

- Eat more pasta and cereals

- Eat more fresh fruit

- Cook vegetables with little or no fat

- Drink skim milk

- Eat nonfat yogurt

- Drink a lot of water

- Read all labels, watching for hidden fat

Dietary Recommendations

Dr. Henry Leis, a breast cancer surgeon, encourages his patients to adopt healthy eating habits for a lifetime. His advice to his breast cancer patients includes:

A low-fat diet is recommended. Other factors of major importance include a high fiber, reduced calorie diet; avoidance of obesity; proper exercise; use of appropriate vitamins and minerals as supplements; limiting consumption of alcohol, salt-cured, smoked and nitrate-cured foods; and reducing levels of environmental carcinogens.

"We are what we eat," and what we eat is one thing we can all control. A sensible approach of reducing dietary fat, adding additional fiber and eating a balanced diet can be a valuable tool in your recovery from breast cancer.

Staying Physically Fit

Recovery after breast cancer is also a time to consider an exercise program that suits you. Your hospital or clinic may offer or recommend exercise classes for breast cancer patients with a focus on regaining the range of motion of the surgical arm. These programs are very beneficial.

While these programs are helpful for your surgical recovery, you should also begin a program of regular exercise. The program you select does not need to be elaborate. You do not need to join a gym or health club to begin. For example, walking is one of the most beneficial exercises. Consider your time and lifestyle to find an exercise that you will enjoy and participate in on a regular basis.

Benefits of Regular Exercise

Whatever exercise you select and consistently do will not only benefit you physically with higher energy levels, but it will also serve to increase your psychological recovery from breast cancer. Exercise has been shown to improve both physical strength and psychological mood. Exercise also reduces pain by promoting the release of natural painkillers referred to as "endorphins" or "natural morphine" into the body. Regular exercise has been proven to help reduce depression.

It is proven that a regular program of walking during breast cancer treatment can significantly increase the quality of life for a patient. However, it is important to get your physician's approval before starting this or any exercise program.

Recommended Walking Exercise Program

Frequency: Four times a week minimum, six times a week maximum; try not to skip more than one day in a row if your health allows.

Goal: Gradually increase and maintain your heart rate at 100 to 120 beats per minute during walking.

Duration: Brisk walking at your own rate; starting at 10 minutes per session and increasing gradually to 30 minutes per session as tolerated.

Place: Preferably outdoors, when weather permits; indoor mall or treadmill.

Attire: Comfortable shoes designed for walking; layered, loose, cotton clothing to absorb perspiration; and personal identification in case of an emergency.

Recommended Routine

1. Five minutes of slow walking to warm up.

2. Increase walking to a brisk pace to increase heart rate to 100 to 120 beats per minute (take your pulse for 6 seconds and multiply by 10 to check your heart rate).

3. Gradually increase the time your pulse remains at your target heart rate by extending your walk as tolerated. Walking should increase your energy after your heart rate returns to normal, without causing fatigue. Do not exercise to a point of causing fatigue; this is not healthy or recommended.

4. For the last five minutes, reduce your pace to allow your heart rate to return to normal gradually.

Do not exercise if you have:

- Fever

- Nausea or vomiting

- Muscle joint pain and swelling

- Bleeding from any source

- Irregular heart beat

- Dizziness or fainting

- Chest, arm or jaw pain

- Intravenous chemotherapy administration on the same day

- Blood drawing on the same day—may exercise afterwards, but prior exercise may alter counts

- Any restrictions placed on exercise activities by a physician

Exercise Precautions During Treatment

If you are receiving chemotherapy, your nurse or physician will alert you if your counts are in a range where exercise is not advised. Ask your nurse when you have your blood drawn if your counts are still in a safe range. **Recommendations of when not to exercise are as follows**:

- White blood count less than 3,000 mm^3

- Absolute granulocyte count less than 2,500 mm^3

- Hemoglobin/hematocrit less than 10g/dl

- Platelet count less than 25,000 mm^3

Exercise During Treatment

Exercise during treatments—chemotherapy or radiation therapy—has to be self-paced. Only you can determine how much you can tolerate and when you feel up to exercising. Begin at a modest level and gradually increase your length of time. Take into consideration that during treatment there may be periods of decreased performance due to effects of treatment. Do not increase your fatigue by pushing yourself during these times.

A walking exercise program can be easily modified to meet your changing needs during treatment; it can be started, suspended, decreased, or accelerated according to your physical energy. You may also want to consider other types of exercise such as biking, swimming or gardening.

Check with your physician to determine if this walking program or any other exercise program is recommended during your recovery. Clinical studies have proven that women who walked four to five times weekly during treatments, for 20 to 45 minutes, had more energy; experienced less depression, nausea and insomnia; gained less weight; and required less medication to control side effects of treatment than women who did not exercise. An exercise program is one thing you can do to promote your own recovery while you are still in treatment.

Beginning an Exercise Program

If you are beginning an exercise program for the first time, check with your physician for approval and recommendations. You may want to ask a friend or a mate to join you in your new venture. Begin to slowly and gradually work up your endurance. Do not push yourself or exhaust your physical reserves; this is not healthy. Instead, look at this as a special time set aside to take care of your own needs and enjoy the activity. The rewards will be increased physical stamina and psychological well-being.

Exercise Tips:

- Walk with a partner, if possible

- Carry identification with you

- Listen to inspirational tapes or your favorite music if you walk alone

- Keep an exercise log or diary to monitor your progress

- Exercise at the same time of day if possible to make walking routine

- Drink a full glass of water before and after you walk

- Walk in a safe area, away from traffic

REMEMBER

Exercise can elevate your mood and increase physical endurance.

Walking is one of the best forms of exercise.

Ask someone to join you; this will increase the likelihood that you will continue the program.

Do not select a diet to lose weight; instead, select a diet to create health.

Diets that limit the amount of food eaten and create hunger are psychologically stressful and should always be avoided.

Watching the amount of fat in your diet can improve your health and may cause a loss of weight.

Do not allow three numbers on a bathroom scale to dictate how you feel about yourself.

Concentrate on healthy eating habits, not numbers on a scale.

Refer to Tearout Worksheets
Exercise Guidelines After Breast Cancer - Page 223
Relaxation Response Guidelines - Page 225

SURVIVORSHIP

Loss in our lives causes us to stop and
review what we have and where we are.
At this point we can learn how we can
grow and how we can make our lives
more rewarding as a result
of the experience.

—*Judy Kneece*

If I had my life to live over . . .
I'd dare to make more mistakes next time.
I'd relax. I would limber up.
I would be sillier than I have been this trip.
I would take fewer things seriously.
I would take more chances.
I would take more trips.
I would climb more mountains
and swim more rivers.
I would eat more ice cream
and less beans . . .

—*Nadine Stair, age 85*

MONITORING YOUR BREASTS AFTER SURGERY

During the first year after your diagnosis, you will spend a lot of time seeing physicians about your surgeries and treatments. They will be monitoring many areas of your health, but there are several areas that you will need to observe yourself. One of these is a breast self-exam (BSE) on the remaining breast and the mastectomy or lumpectomy scar areas.

Many women find it difficult to perform BSE after having cancer. However, it is helpful if you can master this fear. Early detection is your surest weapon against breast cancer. There is a small possibility that you could develop cancer in the other breast or have a recurrence in the remaining breast tissue in a lumpectomy breast or in the scar area of a mastectomy. To keep a vigilant guard on your health, you can check your breast(s) on a regular basis and report any changes to your physician. It is important to remember that women find most of the suspicious lumps and that finding them early greatly increases the chances for a successful treatment.

Some women have found it helpful to have a healthcare provider examine their breast(s) and explain what they feel, assuring them that everything in the breast(s) at this time is a normal finding. This exam gives the assurance needed to start their own program of regular examinations, knowing that the breasts have no known abnormalities and that what they find in the surgical breast is a normal change from breast surgery or radiation therapy.

When to Start Your Breast Self-Exam:

- **Lumpectomy patients** should begin breast self-exam at the completion of radiation therapy or when the incision has healed completely.

- **Mastectomy patients** should begin examination of the surgical site approximately two to three months after surgery. You should carefully examine the scar and surrounding area.

- **Reconstructive surgery** patients should examine the entire reconstruction area, beginning when the incision is completely healed, approximately two to three months after the surgery.

When to Perform Your Exam

It is recommended that women perform breast self-exams on a regular basis. Select a quiet, uninterrupted time when you can concentrate. A breast self-exam is especially important since you have had breast cancer.

- **Menstruating women** should check their breast(s) the last day of the menstrual period or several days past.

- **Post-menopausal** women should check their breast(s) the same day of each month.

- **Women receiving treatment** who are not having a regular menstrual period need to select the same day each month.

How to Learn What is Normal after Surgery

Your goal in breast self-exam is to carefully check your breast(s) to learn what is normal for you. All women's breasts feel differently because of the differences in body tissue and the stimulation of their body's hormones on these tissues. Lumpiness in the breast often results because of hormonal changes in the tissues. This is referred to as **normal nodularity**. After checking your breast(s) regularly, you will discover a normal nodularity pattern in your breast(s). Your goal will then be to check for distinct changes in your breast(s), especially new lumps, and report these changes to your doctor.

Sporadic, shooting pain in a surgical breast is not uncommon in the incision area, especially in breast-conserving surgery. This pain can occur for months. Incision scars may have areas that feel firm to touch, which is caused by scar tissue formation during healing. Areas where drains were inserted may also feel firm. You will need to become familiar with these changes soon after your surgery. This will prevent misinterpretation of these normal post-surgical changes. Very rarely does cancer recur in the incision area the first months after surgery. Your physician can help you distinguish and identify these changes.

Potential Changes in the Radiated Breast:

- Darkening in color of the area (suntanned appearance)

- Edema (swelling) of the breast tissues for up to a year

- Gradual decrease in swelling

- A firmness of the radiated tissues, often feeling lumpy to touch

- Skin thickening, greatest in the area of the nipple and areola in breast conserving surgery

- Slight decrease in size of the radiated breast when edema subsides

- Decreased sensitivity of the breast

It is helpful to become familiar with the normal changes occurring after radiation. Some women feel that applying powder or hand lotion to their hands prior to their self-exam assists in moving their hands freely over the breast tissue.

The exam described below has been taken from the **MammaCare®** method. This method was developed from research at the University of Florida and is now considered state-of-the-art in breast self-exam techniques.

Components of the MammaCare® Exam

Area to Be Examined

The area to be examined is from the middle notch in your collarbone, following under the collarbone until you reach mid-underarm, straight down until you reach your bra line. Follow bra line to middle of breastbone and back to notch. Examine the mastectomy side using the same technique.

The reason for the new, larger boundaries is that the breast is a large gland that covers most of this area, not just the breast mound.

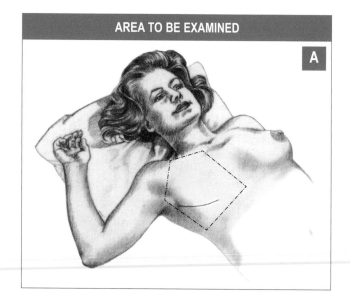

AREA TO BE EXAMINED

A

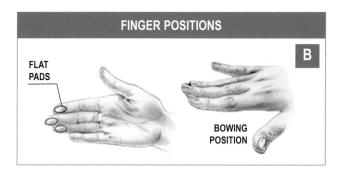

FINGER POSITIONS

FLAT PADS

BOWING POSITION

B

Finger Positions

Use the flats of the three middle fingers, the first joint down to tips. Place flats of fingers in a flat bowing position on the breast tissue.

Pressures

Three levels of pressure will be used when examining each spot on your breast:

Light—barely moves the top layer of skin

Medium—goes halfway through the thickness of the breast

Deep—goes to the base of the breast next to the ribs

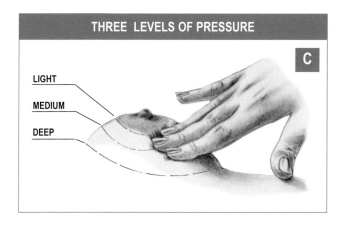

THREE LEVELS OF PRESSURE

LIGHT

MEDIUM

DEEP

C

Do not lift your hand or release the pressure from your breast as you make these three circles.

Using the three levels of pressure allows you to carefully examine the full thickness of the breast and not displace small lumps into fibrous tissues or into your rib area. Pressures do not injure your breast tissue.

Step 1 - Side-Lying Position

Use the following techniques to examine the lumpectomy breast or the mastectomy site:

- Lie down on the bed, roll onto your left side to examine your right breast.

- Pull your knees up slightly, rotate your right shoulder to the flat of the bed.

- Place your right hand, palm up on your forehead. Your nipple should point directly toward the ceiling. Use your left hand to examine your right breast. You may place a small pillow under the arch of the back to increase comfort.

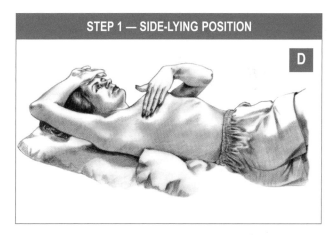

STEP 1 — SIDE-LYING POSITION

D

This position allows you to examine the outer half of the breast by spreading out the tissue. Fifty percent of all cancers occur in the area of the breast which extends from the nipple to underneath the arm. The side-lying position prevents breast tissue from falling into the underarm area.

Step 2 - Side-Lying Exam

- Using the flat pads of your three middle fingers in the bowing position (B), begin your exam under the arm. Make dime-sized circles using the three levels of pressure in each spot (C), following the up and down pattern of search (E). Do not release the pressure as you spiral downward. Ten to 16 vertical strips will be needed. Continue the pattern of search until you reach your nipple.

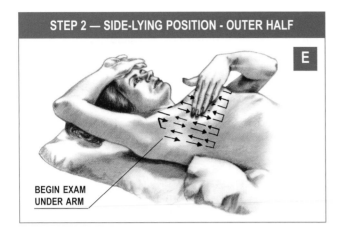

STEP 2 — SIDE-LYING POSITION - OUTER HALF

E

BEGIN EXAM
UNDER ARM

Step 3 - Back-Lying Exam

- When you reach your nipple, roll onto your back; remove your hand from your forehead and place this arm along side your body on the bed (F).

- Continue the exam of the nipple using the same pressures (C). Do not squeeze the nipple.

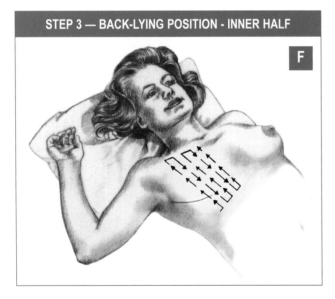

STEP 3 — BACK-LYING POSITION - INNER HALF

F

Report any discharge from your nipple not associated with the onset of a menstrual period, hormonal medications, sexual stimulation or excessive manipulation of the breasts. A bloody discharge or a discharge from only one breast needs to be reported promptly.

- Examine the remaining breast tissue with the same pressures and pattern of search until you reach your breastbone.

Repeat steps 1-3, examining the opposite side.

Step 4 - Lymph Node Exam

- Make a row of circles above and below your collarbone.

- While standing, check the depressed area near your neck by rolling your shoulders upward, and turning your face toward the side you are examining. With the opposite hand, place your fingers in the formed depression and check carefully.

- Feel under each arm for axillary lymph node enlargement.

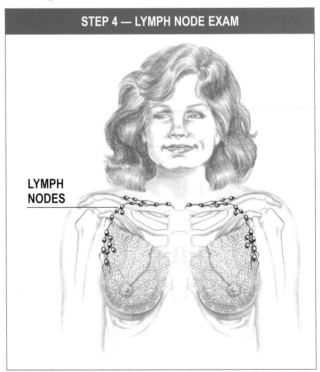

STEP 4 — LYMPH NODE EXAM

LYMPH
NODES

Lymph nodes are soft to hard, pea-like areas in the lymphatic system. They may become enlarged from cancer or infection. Enlarged lymph nodes do not always indicate cancer. Report any lymph node enlargement to your healthcare provider.

Step 5 - Visual Exam

A visual inspection of your breast(s) is important. Some cancers do not form a hard lump. The first indication of cancer may be one you can see and not feel. Looking into a mirror, closely examine your breast(s) in the four positions shown below:

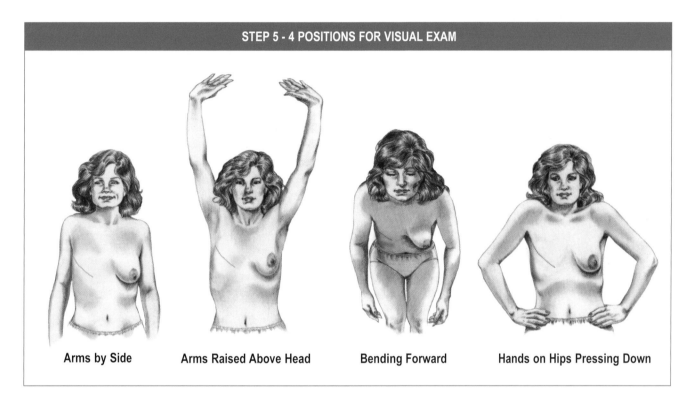

STEP 5 - 4 POSITIONS FOR VISUAL EXAM

| Arms by Side | Arms Raised Above Head | Bending Forward | Hands on Hips Pressing Down |

Carefully observe your incision. It is normal for it to be raised and red in the beginning. The color will gradually begin to fade to a light pink and the scar area will flatten out. A lumpectomy scar area may have a depression or sinking in of the tissues. Look for the following changes in the remaining tissues surrounding your scar and the non-surgical breast:

- Texture of your skin for an orange peel appearance

- Color changes in breast tissues

- Swelling or decreased size of the non-radiated breast

- Dimpling, bulging or pulling in of the skin

- Inverted nipple (not normally inverted)

- Crusty material or irritation around nipple

- Open sore or bump

- Difference in vein pattern over one breast (much larger veins or increased number of veins in one breast)

Breast Visual Exam

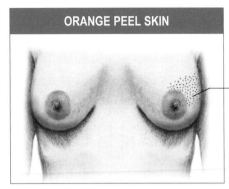

ORANGE PEEL SKIN

- Texture of your skin—may appear like an orange peeling

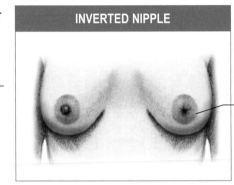

INVERTED NIPPLE

- Inverted nipple—inversion of previously normal nipple

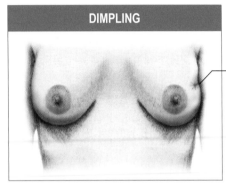

DIMPLING

- Dimpling or pulling in of the skin

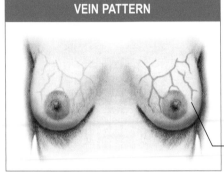

VEIN PATTERN

- Difference in vein pattern on one breast — much larger veins or increased number of veins

Mammograms After Surgery

Mammograms, on a regular schedule, are an important part of monitoring your breast(s). After a diagnosis of breast cancer it is very important that the lumpectomy breast and remaining breast be monitored with mammography. If you had bilateral mastectomies, a prophylactic mastectomy or reconstruction, ask your physician for recommendations concerning regular mammograms. Some physicians may require more frequent mammograms for lumpectomy and mastectomy patients the first several years. Other physicians feel yearly mammography is adequate surveillance. Your physician will tell you what schedule you will follow. Remember, even if you are under 35, your doctor may now want you to go for your mammograms on a yearly basis. Remind your doctor if your annual checkup does not include a mammogram. Remember to schedule your mammogram when your breast(s) is least tender. This is at the end of your period if you are pre-menopausal.

Make sure that your mammography facility has been certified by the U.S. Food and Drug Administration (FDA) for having met quality standards.

Preparation for Mammogram

When you go for a mammogram, do not wear deodorant, perfume or powder on your upper body, as this could appear as a shadow or spot on your mammogram film. If you have had a painful mammogram in the past, stop caffeine intake several days prior or ask your physician about taking ibuprofen to reduce discomfort.

If you change facilities for your mammogram, be sure to take your previous films for comparison. If you move, call and ask to pick up your old mammography films to take to your new provider. This is an important part of your health record and it is necessary for a new physician to have prior mammography films in order to compare your new films to your past for small changes. Some facilities will call and have your films sent to the new provider after you sign a release. If you schedule an appointment at a new facility and have not moved your previous films, you need to call so that your new provider will have the previous films at the time they read your new films.

REMEMBER

Breast self-exam is a valuable tool
for monitoring for local recurrence.

When you complete your monthly
exam, congratulate yourself
for taking an active part
in guarding your health.
Then forget about it
until next month.

Have a mammogram yearly.

Practice breast self-exam monthly.

Have a healthcare provider do a clinical
exam at least yearly or more often,
if necessary.

Using these three methods will help
assure that a vigilant watch is being
kept over your continued good health.
You need to practice all three
methods of detection.

Fear of recurrence is the
number one fear of cancer patients.
This is a natural reaction after a diagnosis.
However, we must not allow ourselves
to be controlled by our fear of tomorrow.
The cure for fear is to name what is
causing it and to face it,
whatever it may be.
Pushing ourselves to move
through our fear is the first step
to claiming peace and to
enhancing our life.

—Judy Kneece

When our only reference is the past
we may not see or experience what
is actually happening today.
If we drove our automobiles using the
rearview mirror as our only reference point
we would probably crash quickly.
If we want to successfully drive a car,
we must see more than what is behind us.
This is true for directing our lives as well.
The past should only serve as one
of many reference points.

—Judy Tatelbaum

MONITORING YOUR FUTURE HEALTH FOR RECURRENCE

The end of your treatment is finally here. This is the day that you have been waiting for since your diagnosis. When it comes, however, you may be feeling a little anxious, perhaps even a little frightened, and certainly wondering what to expect in the future. You've probably heard about and met women who have remained cancer free for many years. But you've probably also heard about women whose breast cancer recurred, sometimes within months or years after they finished treatment. This is obviously terrifying for you and your family.

Now that you are no longer in active treatment, it is important to know how to monitor your health in partnership with your healthcare team. You need to understand what to expect in the future months and years when you return for your checkups and to also know the signs and symptoms that should be reported to your physician between visits. This is vital because most recurrent breast cancer is suspected or found by women themselves, and the majority of recurrences are detected between scheduled medical visits. When choosing the doctor to handle your follow-up care, consider choosing the one with whom you feel most comfortable and one that is an expert in cancer treatment.

Signs and Symptoms to Report

Certain symptoms may indicate that your breast cancer has recurred. If you experience any of these symptoms, it is important to call your doctor so that they can be evaluated and appropriate follow-up diagnostic tests performed. Symptoms that need to be reported to your physician include:

- Chronic bone pain or tenderness in an area

- Skin rashes, redness, or chronic swelling

- New lumps in your breast, chest wall, under arm or on the neck

- Changes in your breast(s) or surgical site such as a rash or discoloration

- Chest pain and any shortness of breath

- Persistent abdominal pain or abdominal swelling

- Headaches, dizziness, or rapid changes in vision

- Changes in weight, especially weight loss

The most common ways recurrence is discovered is by women reporting changes or symptoms as described above, followed by a physician's interview about recent physical history at a follow-up appointment, and finally by a physician's physical exam of a patient. The majority of breast cancer recurrences happen within the first five years. Therefore, one of the most important things you can do is keep your scheduled return appointments and maintain open, honest communication with your healthcare team by reporting any changes you observe in your health. With this open partnership, any recurrence should be detected early.

Monitoring Your Health

Breast Self Exam: Perform a breast self-exam (BSE) each month. This includes a careful check of your breast(s) or surgical site for any new lumps, redness, or swelling. This is particularly important if you have had breast surgery of any kind (mastectomy, with or without reconstruction or implant, or lumpectomy). If you do not feel competent performing a self-exam, your healthcare provider can instruct you on how to do a correct exam. You will then be able to tell the difference between a lump, normal breast tissue, normal scar tissue, changes in a radiated breast and implant material.

Follow-Up Exams: Have a thorough physical exam every three to six months for the first three years after your primary therapy then every six to 12 months for the next two years; and annually thereafter. Close follow-up during the first few years is important because 60 to 80 percent of all breast cancer recurrences are detected within the first three years after therapy. Of course, your physician will have you come back into the office between visits if you notice any change. Your healthcare provider will take a detailed medical history at each visit. During your physical exam, your doctor will look for any physical changes that relate to your general health and/or any symptoms that may suggest your cancer has recurred or has spread to another part of your body (systemic disease). In addition to performing a careful breast exam, your doctor will closely examine your entire chest wall and check for lymph node enlargement in other areas of your body. Your heart and lungs will be listened to and your abdomen, neck, and other areas will be checked for any swelling. Your doctor will also check for any changes in neurological abnormalities, liver enlargement, or bone tenderness that may be a sign of metastasis.

If you are in good physical condition and have no symptoms, a physical exam and a blood count may be all the diagnostic testing required at your follow-up visits. However, if your physician feels it is necessary, other tests (see Appendix A for complete descriptions) that may be performed.

Potential Diagnostic Tests:

- Chest x-ray

- Bone scan

- Ultrasound of liver

- Computed tomography scan (CT or CAT) of areas of concern

- Breast cancer tumor markers CA15.3, CA27.29 and CEA.

Remember, however, one of the most important components of the exam will be your reporting any changes or symptoms you have experienced.

- **Mammography After Breast Surgery:** Have a yearly mammogram. If you had breast-conserving therapy (lumpectomy), you should have your first post-treatment mammogram six months after completion of radiation therapy, then annually, or as indicated by your doctor. (Some physicians keep the six-month schedule for the lumpectomy patients for several years.) If you have had a mastectomy, you still need to have a mammogram of the remaining breast. Some physicians may also prescribe a mammogram of the tissue remaining at the site of the mastectomy while some may order a mammogram if you have an implant(s).

- **Pelvic Exam:** Every woman should have a pelvic exam at regular intervals. For most women, this will be yearly. If you have had a total abdominal hysterectomy and oophorectomy (removal of your ovaries), this may be done less often. Your periodic pelvic exams should include a Pap test as well as rectal and vaginal exams. If you take or have taken tamoxifen, you could be at increased risk for endometrial (uterine) cancer and, therefore, your physician will ask you specifically about vaginal discharge or bleeding. There is no need for routine endometrial biopsies as was once recommended.

■ **Bone Density Scan:** Treatment with chemotherapy for breast cancer accelerates the loss of bone density the first year after treatment. Decreased bone density puts one at higher risk for osteoporosis, a bone thinning disease that can increase the risk for bone fractures. The most common sites for fractures are the hips, spine, and wrists. However, osteoporosis causes progressive bone loss throughout the skeleton causing fractures in any site. Osteoporosis can be difficult to fight because it is a silent disease. It is often missed until a person suffers a fracture.

Bone density testing is a safe, non-invasive radiological procedure that helps determine if individuals have a bone density level that puts them at risk for osteoporosis or strongly suggests that they have osteoporosis. The recommended standard today is the <u>d</u>ual <u>e</u>nergy <u>x</u>-ray <u>a</u>bsorptiometry (DEXA) measurement of the spine and hip. It is suggested that all women over the age of 50 and all women completing breast cancer treatment have a DEXA to measure their bone density. Bone density tests of other sites of the body such as the wrist and heel are less accurate because they are screening tests, not diagnostic procedures like DEXA. If a screening test indicates low bone mass, a DEXA should be ordered to determine true bone loss. Screening tests should never be used as a follow-up to measure improvement in bone density. A score of minus 1 to minus 2 indicates osteopenia (some bone loss), a condition that can lead to osteoporosis. A value of minus 2 (some use minus 2.5) or greater shows osteoporosis. Osteoporosis has no cure, but women diagnosed with the condition and their healthcare providers can usually develop a treatment plan that includes:

■ Diet adequate in calcium and Vitamin D

■ Appropriate physical activity

■ Review of any medications they are taking that can cause bone loss

■ Regular visits for counseling and check-ups

■ Medications to prevent or preserve additional bone loss (Fosamax®, Miacalcin®, Evista® and Actonel®)

■ Estrogen replacement therapy can be used, but may not be an appropriate choice after breast cancer

REMEMBER

Remember to write down any questions to ask your physician before your follow-up visit.

Your understanding of what to report and when is an essential part of monitoring your health.

You are still human and will have aches and pains.

Don't ignore persistent symptoms. Report them to your healthcare provider and let them determine their significance.

Keep your scheduled appointments.

Communicate openly with your healthcare team.

The fact is there is no way
to rewrite our past.
What has happened has happened.
Acceptance is the only way to
make peace with our past and move
on after a cancer diagnosis.

Our goal should be to become
designers of our future life.
We need to plan to add to our life
things or events that make us smile,
inspire us to keep going, and let us
experience a deep, inner sense of peace.
What do you plan to add to
your life in the future?

A major sign of emotional recovery
is when we reach out to help others
in need. It is in serving others that
we rediscover our worth as a
human being and recapture
the best we can be.

Helping other people is a
powerful secret for healing ourselves.

—Judy Kneece

FACING THE FUTURE
AFTER BREAST CANCER

"I consider myself a survivor, not a victim. I think about recurrence, but it no longer consumes me. I do not fear death, nor do I fear life after having had breast cancer. My life will never be the same as before, but any negatives breast cancer has brought have been matched by positives."

HARRIETT BARRINEAU
SURVIVOR

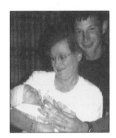

"I remember that while I was still in the hospital I said to my mother-in-law that I needed to find out why this had happened to me. I know she thought I was looking to place blame. But I was really looking for meaning. Somehow, after struggling with all the normal emotions and asking 'why,' I finally arrived at the inner feeling that I had been given the gift of being diagnosed with breast cancer—yes, a gift! But I had to do something to make this a reality. So I changed careers, got involved in local breast cancer causes, and joined the Young Survival Coalition. Now I am 'fighting for our future' and working to ensure the quality and quantity of the lives of young women affected by breast cancer. Everyday, I am on the front lines seeing that others have the tools they need to negotiate their own diagnosis. My life is extremely fulfilling and emotionally rewarding."

ANNA CLUXTON
SURVIVOR

"My husband and I are thankful for the experience. It has brought us moments of tenderness and closeness that we might never have otherwise experienced. We have been through so much that we feel like we have lived a lifetime together already. Fortunately, we still have a long life ahead of us too."

No woman would ever choose to have breast cancer. Breast cancer changes your life, and there are some things that will never be the same after your diagnosis. Yet, many have shared that the breast cancer experience added a new dimension to their lives—one that allowed them to enjoy life even more than before. If you are reading this chapter shortly after your diagnosis, you may find this unbelievable. However, as time passed and side effects subsided, many women found that their diagnosis presented an opportunity to reevaluate their lives and make positive changes that they had postponed because they were waiting for the right time. Take it from others who have survived. Now is the right time to look at your life closely and start to live the life that you have always wanted.

Recovery Timetable

Recovery from breast cancer is a gradual process mentally, just as it is physically. The physical healing usually comes long before the psychological healing. Physicians and your healthcare team focus on your physical healing. However, you must manage your psychological recovery on your own timetable. Some women are eager to put the experience behind them, while others need time to absorb the impact of the changes that cancer brings. Only you can decide what is best for you. Just as your treatment team has plans for you to recover physically, **you need to chart a mental recovery plan**. You need to plan how you will deal with future fears and life decisions.

Survivorship Attitudes

In my work with breast cancer survivors, I have listened to hundreds of breast cancer stories. As a caregiver who intervened throughout the entire breast cancer experience, I shared their tears, fears and triumphs. From all of this I have observed what I feel are survivorship attitudes that can help build an even richer life after a breast cancer diagnosis. These attitudes are not new. There are no secrets revealed here. Yet, somehow in the midst of a crisis it can be helpful if someone reminds you of what has worked in the past for others who have encountered a similar experience.

Survivorship attitudes led to happiness in spite of the event that paid an unexpected visit to their lives. Survivorship attitudes do not deny the loss and pain you endured, but rather encompass the loss as a learning and motivating experience. Breast cancer survivors have used these lessons to make changes in their life, including taking care of themselves emotionally and physically. As you read through this list, think of how these attitudes may help to add a sense of control and joy back to your life.

Tips from Survivors
Understand Your Cancer and Treatment

- Demystify cancer. Learn the facts about cancer. Correct your misconceptions. Cancer is a scary word and experience. However, because a cancer is unique to each person, you have to learn the details of your own cancer, treatment and recovery plan to correct misconceptions and move forward with correct facts.

- Participate in your treatment decisions. Get answers to your questions before you agree to surgery or treatments. This is your life and your breast(s), and you will feel much more in control when you express your needs regarding treatment decisions. Refer to the tear out worksheets to find the questions that are specific to each physician involved in your care. Ask the questions you choose. Answering your questions about your treatment is part of a physician's responsibility. This is the beginning of your own recovery, participating in decisions about your body.

- Form a partnership with your treatment team in battling the disease. Learn how you can best participate for maximum response during treatment. Communicate openly and honestly with your treatment team. They need your input. Remember, you are the only one that knows what is really happening to your body and what tools you need to recover.

Dealing with Emotions and Fears

- Do not suppress your emotions. Cry when you need to, and talk about your experience. Grieve over your loss. This is not a sign of emotional weakness; it is a normal response to a loss in life. Talk to someone you can trust about your feelings and fears. It may be necessary to find this person outside of the family unit—a professional counselor or peer.

- Identify your fears. Write them down and take action to disarm them. Fear is a paralyzing factor. Our fears rob us of peace in the moment and torment us about decisions in the future. It can only be mastered by naming the fear and taking action to face them with action.

Making Peace with The Past

- Do not concentrate on the "what ifs." Thinking about what you could or could not have done differently will not change anything. The past is the past, and yesterday cannot be changed. Some people get emotionally stuck trying to figure out "why." When I was young I would ask my dad "why"? He would look at me and smile and say, "All I know is that it is part of life and we may never know why." In the field of breast cancer, we don't know "why" most women have breast cancer. Only those with the BRCA mutated genes have absolute answers of why. So, concentrate on what you can do now that it has happened rather than "why it happened."

The Hidden Roadblocks of Recovery

In emotional recovery there are unseen attitudes that can sabotage your mental recovery. These attitudes are often not seen by others but are mentally engulfing. Feeling like a victim, anger, hate and bitterness are sabotagers of your recovery. These emotions are all "joy robbers." Allowing the diagnosis of breast cancer to cause you to be angry because you feel unfairly victimized will rob you of your ability to get on with life and plan and find the happiness you deserve. Let it go. Refuse to let it use any of your energy or occupy your thoughts. Don't live in the yesterdays of your life. Live today—it is the only time you can impact or change.

In his book *Life Strategies: Doing What Works, Doing What Matters*, Dr. Phil McGraw sums up the impact of feeling like a victim of circumstance:

> *By convincing yourself that you are a victim, you are guaranteed to have no progress, no healing and no victory. Your flight from responsibility will prevent you from taking the bit in your teeth and going to work to control your life. If you truly want change, and you truly acknowledge that you create your own experience, then you must analyze what you've done or haven't done to create the undesirable results. . . . If in any part of your life, you are angry, hurt, or upset in any way, then you choose those feelings and are accountable for their presence in your life. . . . Bottom line: You are not a victim . . . you are creating the emotions that flow from those situations. . . . However difficult or unusual it may seem, embrace the fact that you own the problem . . . While everybody else is out there blaming those who aren't responsible for the results in their life you can be as on target as a laser-guided missile, and, therefore, work on those things that can truly change your life. That gives you a tremendous head start in the solution category.*

Plan to turn loose all anger, bitterness and hatred toward people and events in the past; this frees you to use your time constructively to live today and build a better tomorrow.

Replace unhealthy attitudes with those that lay a foundation for health—love, peace and joy. Dr. Herbert Benson of Harvard Medical School says "It is strongly suggested that you could use your mind to change your physiology in a beneficial way, improve your health, and perhaps reduce your need for medications." Our thoughts create the chemical environment of our body. What we think about is powerful, and affects our feelings, which in turn affect our behaviors and vice versa.

Thoughts are the birthplace of our feelings. Feelings then lead to behaviors.

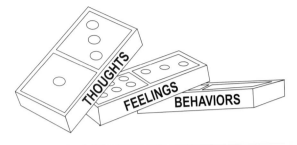

Know that you may not be able to choose what happens to your body but that you can choose what happens in your mind. Be the master of your thoughts and refuse to camp in the land of despair and hopelessness. Negative thoughts are normal, but you can choose to acknowledge them and take steps to think on more positive aspects of your life. There is an old saying: "We can't help it if birds fly over our head, but we can stop them from building a nest." When you recognize a thought as negative and it is dragging your spirit down with worry, acknowledge it and decide to deliberately think about something that is pleasant to you. Learn focused thinking. **Do not focus** on things that you have **no power over or cannot change**. Ask yourself, can I change this or influence it by what I am thinking? If not, concentrate on the things that you have control over and can change. You can decide what thoughts you allow to "build a nest" in your mind: choose hope, think about things that make your spirit smile, pray, think gratefully about what others have done for you, think lovingly.

Acknowledge that there are going to be days when things don't go well and you won't feel well physically or psychologically. But remember to reach out, ask for help if you need it, and know that this, too, will pass. Don't try to be a superwoman.

Prepare yourself for those emotionally trying days (of treatment, medical tests or anniversary dates) with a physically and emotionally stress-free schedule as often as possible. Recruit a friend to share this time or plan a special treat for yourself to soften the experience.

"Choosing thoughts contributes to your experiences, because when you choose your thoughts, you choose consequences that are associated with those thoughts. If you choose thoughts that demean and depreciate you, then you choose the consequences of low self-esteem and low self-confidence. If you choose thoughts contaminated with anger and bitterness, then you will create an experience of alienation, isolation, and hostility. . . . There's a very powerful connection at work here. Your physiology determines your energy and action level. If your internal dialogue is negative and self-effacing, then the physiology that simultaneously occurs will be just as negative. Your depressed thoughts suppress energy and action. Your body will conform to that central computer message. You are mentally, behaviorally, and physiology programming yourself to go through life in a particular way."

—Dr. Phil McGraw
Life Strategies: Doing What Works, Doing What Matters

Places to Find Encouragement

- Participate in a support group. Find a group that provides education as well as support. Women who attend support groups tend to adjust better than those who do not reach out.

- Use your spiritual faith as a source of strength and a place to find answers and give meaning to the hard questions of life.

- Allow your family and friends to participate in your recovery by helping you. Tell them what you need. Don't make them guess. It is therapeutic for them to feel needed.

- Find outside support resources for your family, such as written materials and support groups, to help them understand and adjust to your diagnosis. Encourage them to reach out for their own sources of support.

Share Your Gratefulness

- Stop long enough to say "thank you" or "I appreciate you" to your caregivers, whether they are the healthcare staff, family or friends. Like you, they need to know they are appreciated and valued. Being a care-giver is not always easy, and most people forget to share what they feel.

Diet and Exercise

- Eat healthy, exercise regularly, rest when you need to, and get enough sleep. These are the foundations for physical and emotional health.

- Don't resort to covering your anxiety with alcohol or recreational drugs. This only postpones your psychological recovery and can lead to depression.

Monitoring Your Health

- Follow your physician's guide for medical monitoring after cancer. Keep your appointments, perform breast self-exam monthly, get your mammograms, but **don't** make a "career" out of cancer. Don't let it dominate your thoughts and actions.

Your Life Plan

- Take time to do the things that make you feel good, whatever they may be. Plan your own fun times. Don't wait for happiness to come. Go and find it!

- Decide when and what you are going to do to make this a time of intensive personal growth. Chart new courses for yourself—take a class, read a long book, take a trip, plant a flower garden or whatever you have always wanted to do "when I have time." This will give you new energy and facilitate recovery.

You must be willing to say, 'I know it may be scary for a while, but I am worth it. I'm going to stop denying myself of getting my goals and dreams. I am going to set goals, make a strategy and take action.' . . . Decide that you are going to move onward and upward. Make a life decision to risk reasonably, risk responsibility, but risk. I'm not talking about sky-diving here. I'm talking about letting yourself want more and taking the action to get it.

Dr. Phil McGraw

Surround yourself with the things you love . . . music, books, pets, hobbies, whatever makes you smile. You deserve it.

The Final Step of Recovery

From my experience, I know a person has made peace with what has happened in their life when they decide to give back to others out of their own experience. They offer their support to others who are traveling the same unknown path of a cancer diagnosis. Many women can benefit and gain support from your learning experience during breast cancer treatment. Find the best expression for your talents. Consider becoming a *Reach To Recovery* volunteer and help other patients or participate in fundraisers or activities to support other patients. Find your way to pass on the support you received.

Look at the breast cancer experience as the "caution light" in your life that allowed you to slow down and examine your real needs and wishes for the future.

It is vital to remember that you are **not** a **statistic of breast cancer**. You are an individual. Do not look at your future purely through statistics. If only one person has ever beaten the odds, you have the right to become the second.

Survivorship is mostly attitude—the attitude that "I CAN." Become the best survivor ever! Start today to build the tomorrow that you desire.

Breast cancer is an unwelcome visitor in any woman's life. You have found yourself forced to embrace an enemy. Yet, even in the midst of this frightening and often lonely experience, you do have the capacity to find new strength and work through the challenge. Like thousands of other women, you can become a triumphant survivor.

My love and best wishes for a happy and healthy future.

Judy

Refer to Tearout Worksheet
Personal Plan for Recovery - Page 227

The caterpillar views the cocoon as life threatening . . .
The butterfly views the cocoon as life-giving . . .

A cancer diagnosis is similar to the transformation of a caterpillar into a butterfly. At diagnosis, as a little caterpillar crawling along in life, you find yourself physically coming to a stopping place during treatment where you spin a cocoon around your body. Inside this safe web you hibernate physically and emotionally. However, during this time, a strange phenomenon is occurring—strangely enough you are changing your very essence.

Just like the caterpillar, after a period of dormancy, your treatments end—the cocoon breaks open. You emerge, a new and beautiful person—just like the butterfly. To your amazement, you can now fly! Time spent in the cocoon has transformed you.

No longer do you crawl but now you can fly in a newfound freedom. You may not even recognize your former self. From your vantage point, you enjoy life from a new perspective. Your freedom brings joy into others' lives as they view your brilliance, and confidence as you spread your new wings. They are attracted by and amazed at the change they see in you. Peers look to you as a role model. You have emerged as a new creature, my dear one.

Cancer, though one of the scariest words you will ever hear, is surprisingly preparing you for an even better life. So use your time in the cocoon of treatment as a time to redefine yourself and your life. Your challenge is to live each day to its fullest. You are being set free to fly!

UNDERSTANDING DIAGNOSTIC TESTS

Blood Counts

Your doctor will monitor your blood counts by drawing blood from your finger, arm or implanted vascular port on a regular basis. This blood test evaluates how you respond to the effects of chemotherapy, monitors for infections and detects changes in your blood chemistry. The main counts monitored will be:

- **Red blood cells (RBCs)**—carry oxygen to all parts of your body

- **White blood cells (WBCs)**—combat infection and provide immunity

- **Platelets**—determine how your blood will clot

- **Electrolytes** (potassium, magnesium, sodium, chloride, glucose and carbon dioxide)

- **Hemoglobin** (iron)—the portion of the red blood cells (RBCs) that attaches to oxygen

Remind the technician drawing the sample not to use your surgical arm. If you had bilateral mastectomies, the technician will need to use sterile procedures to reduce the potential for infection.

Normal Values	
Red blood cells (RBCs)	4.2-5.4 million/mm^3
White blood cells (WBCs)	5,000-10,000 /mm^3
Hemoglobin (Hgb)	12-16 g/dl
Platelets	150,000-400,000/mm^3

Bone Scan

Your physician may order a bone scan after your diagnosis. This scan is one of the most commonly performed nuclear medicine procedures used to determine if cancer has spread to the bones. The test is routinely ordered by physicians to stage your cancer.

On the day of the scan, you will have a radioactive substance intravenously injected into your arm, similar to having your blood drawn. This will cause little discomfort, and no side effects should occur from the injected material. In order for the radioactive substance to get to the bone, you will have a wait of several hours (one to three) before beginning the actual testing. You will need to drink several glasses of water after your injection to help eliminate, through your kidneys, any of the substance not picked up by the bones. You may want to take something to read, or you may leave and come back to the clinic for the scan. There is no other preparation on your part.

The scan requires you to lie on a table while a machine moves above your body from head to toe. You will be asked to empty your bladder before the test. You will be dressed, and there is no discomfort unless you find it difficult to lie flat and still. The scan may require as long as one hour to complete. The machine will scan your body and produce images of the structure of your bones. This machine does not give off radiation to your body. The only radiation you receive is in the injected substance, which is equal to the amount of radiation received from a regular diagnostic x-ray. An increased amount of the radioactive substance in an area of the bones, referred to as a "hot spot," may indicate an abnormality that the physician will further evaluate.

The radioactive substance given is of insufficient radioactivity to necessitate taking any special radiation precautions. The radioactive material will be excreted through the urine within 24 hours. You are not a risk to your family members during this time. The information gathered by the scan will be translated into x-ray pictures and a report will be sent to your physician.

Computed Tomography (CT) Scan

The CT scan, an advanced x-ray technique, enables your physician and the radiologist to view the bones and organs of your head and body in fine detail. This diagnostic procedure allows an earlier and faster diagnosis than the traditional x-ray. The test is performed inside a large x-ray tube. Pictures are taken in rapid sequence and sent to a computer to be studied by the physician and the radiologist.

The part of your body to be examined determines how you will need to prepare for the scan. In some cases, you may be asked not to eat or drink anything prior to the test. You may be given a contrast agent (radioactive substance) to drink, or it may be injected into your vein to help highlight certain body parts. Tell the technologist if you have been given a contrast agent before; if you are allergic to seafood, iodine or other medications; if you have kidney problems; if you are diabetic; or if you are pregnant.

You will be asked to lie very still on a table for the duration of the scan. A built-in communications system enables two-way conversation between you and the technologist at any time during the scan. The automated table will move you into the scanner's x-ray tube, a donut-shaped ring, to take pictures of your body. You can expect to hear mechanical noises from the scanner as it takes pictures and collects data.

Inform your physician if you are claustrophobic. A medication may be given prior to the test to relax you during the scan. If you receive medication, you will need to bring a family member or a friend to drive you home. If you have difficulty lying down and being still because of pain, you may wish to take pain medication prior to the scan.

If you are given a contrast agent, it will naturally leave your body within 24 hours. You should increase the amount of water you drink to help get rid of the agent from your body through your kidneys. CT scans give off no more radiation than a series of regular x-ray studies, and you are not radioactive. This is a painless procedure.

Liver Scan

A liver scan allows your physician to check for structural changes in your liver. Prior to the test, you will be injected with a radioactive contrast agent through a vein. The contrast agent travels to the liver and allows special pictures to be taken, showing the uptake of the contrast agent. Approximately 30 minutes after the agent is administered, you will lie down on a table while a special instrument, a gamma ray detector (Geiger counter), is passed over your abdomen. You will be asked to change positions so all surfaces of the liver can be seen. The gamma ray detector will record the uptake of the contrast agent in the liver, and pictures will be made of the liver. Your physician will then study these pictures.

The contrast agent will naturally leave your body in hours. You are not exposed to large amounts of radioactive material in this test. After the test is completed, you may resume your normal activities. This scanning procedure is completely painless.

Vacuum Assisted Breast Biopsy (Mammotome® or MIBB)

A vacuum assisted breast biopsy refers to the type of biopsy probe used to obtain tissue samples for diagnosis. This procedure is performed in a breast center or in a physician's office. The biopsy requires only a 1/4" skin incision in the breast for insertion of the biopsy probe. This is a minimally invasive biopsy procedure that uses stereotactic or ultrasound images to guide the biopsy probe. A vacuum assisted biopsy can be performed in less than one hour under a local anesthetic, minimizing discomfort.

The advantage of the Mammotome® biopsy is that it is capable of sampling a variety of breast abnormalities such as microcalcifications, asymmetric (unusually shaped) densities (thickenings), solid masses, or nodules. It can obtain multiple tissue samples with one insertion where other methods require multiple insertions of the biopsy device.

If the procedure is being guided with ultrasound, the patient lies on her back or possibly her side. In stereotactic procedures, the patient lies face down on a biopsy table with the breast protruding through an opening. The breast is lightly compressed to immobilize it. This table is similar to the mammogram table that allows the physician to get a clear mammographic image of the area to be sampled. The table is connected to a computer that processes digital images. Placement of the sampling device is guided by a computerized system using x-rays.

While the physician looks at the images using ultrasound or stereotactic, the biopsy probe is inserted into the breast and aligned with the breast abnormality. The probe has a vacuum system that when activated, suctions the tissue into the probe. A rotating cutting device captures the breast tissue and the sample is carried through the probe to a tissue collection area outside the breast. The physician then rotates the probe to the next position to collect additional samples without having to remove and reinsert the probe. The sequence is repeated until all desired areas have been sampled.

When the physician has taken the needed biopsy samples, a small stainless steel tissue marker may be placed in the biopsy site for future monitoring of the exact location. This small maker is undetectable to the patient and allows more accurate follow-up on future mammograms. The biopsy probe is removed from the breast, pressure is applied, and a small bandage is placed over the biopsy area. The tissue samples are sent to a laboratory for analysis by a pathologist. The pathology report is sent to your physician.

Magnetic Resonance Imaging (MRI)

Breast MRI

Breast MRI may be used to more closely evaluate breast abnormalities first seen on a mammogram. Mammography uses low dose x-rays to image the breast while MRI uses powerful magnetic fields. MRI may be used to study the extent of the breast cancer after a diagnosis. Breast cancer can be multi-focal (in more than one area of the breast) but difficult to see on a mammogram; therefore, a physician may want to evaluate both breasts carefully before lumpectomy surgery.

MRI is useful in helping to determine whether breast cancer has spread into the chest wall. If there is evidence of breast cancer in the chest wall, the patient may undergo chemotherapy before surgery. Physicians can also use MRI to detect recurrences in women who have already been treated for breast cancer with lumpectomy.

It is also used to examine implants to see if they are intact or leaking and to further evaluate whether the cancer has spread within the breast or to surrounding areas. MRI also allows physicians to easily visualize the muscle and chest wall in the vicinity of the breast along with the breast tissue. Recently, researchers have studied MRI as a screening tool for women who are at high risk for breast cancer, are young or have dense breasts.

Benefits of MRI:

- Highly sensitive to small lesions

- Effective in visualizing dense breasts

- Evaluation of inverted nipples for evidence of cancer

- Evaluation of the extent of breast cancer

- Visualization of breast implants and ruptures

- Detection of breast cancer recurrence (return) after breast conserving therapy

- Characterization or identification of small lesions missed by mammography

- May be useful in screening women at high risk for breast cancer

MRI Exam:

- The patient lies face down on a special padded table with the breasts falling through openings in the table (no compression is used). The table contains special MRI coils (antenna) that receive the imaging data during the exam.

- A series of images are taken while the patient lies still.

- A tapping sound is heard coming from the machine during the MRI exam.

- The exam typically takes between 30 and 60 minutes.

Preparation for Exam:

- Inform your physician if you think you will have difficulty lying still on your abdomen.

- There is no pain or compression during the exam.

Methylene Blue Dye Localization

This procedure may be required when a suspicious area on a mammogram cannot be felt by the surgeon. The dye is inserted into the suspicious area of the breast to color the area in order to aid the surgeon with the procedure. Using x-ray as a guide, the radiologist inserts the dye by injection with a needle. The surgeon removes the tissue stained by the dye. The tissue is sent to pathology for analysis. Needle localization biopsy or methylene blue are two procedures used to help the surgeon locate suspicious areas during surgery.

Needle Localization Biopsy

Needle localization biopsy is needed when a suspicious place shows up on a mammogram and cannot be felt with the hands. You will be taken to x-ray, where the radiologist will place your breast under a mammography machine. While the breast is visualized, the radiologist will insert a wire into the spot that was seen previously on your mammogram. The insertion of the wire can be uncomfortable, however, analgesic medications can be given to alleviate the discomfort. The wire will be taped to your chest after a series of pictures confirm accurate

placement. You will then be taken to surgery for the removal of the suspicious area. The removed tissue will be sent to the pathologist for diagnosis.

Stereotactic Needle Biopsy

If a suspicious area, that cannot be felt or is very small is seen on a mammogram, stereotactic breast biopsy (Mammotest) may be used to biopsy the area. This biopsy procedure is performed using a mammography table, a biopsy needle and the guidance of a computer. This test, an alternative to surgical biopsy, is done without the discomfort, risk of disfigurement and expense of surgery. The procedure takes approximately 45 minutes to perform, and most patients return to their normal activities within a few hours.

Your breast will be compressed with a special mammography machine while stereo x-ray pictures are taken at angles. After the suspicious area has been identified, the radiologist enters information into a computer that calculates where the needle should be inserted. The area of the breast to be biopsied is deadened with a local anesthetic. An instrument moves the biopsy needle in position and at a rapid rate of speed removes a sample of the suspicious tissue. Because stereotactic biopsy uses a needle, damage to nearby tissue is minimal, unlike surgery, which may cause scarring to the breast. When the biopsy is complete, a small bandage will be placed over the biopsy site, and you may return to your normal activities. You may shower the same day of the biopsy.

The biopsy sample will be sent to the pathology lab for evaluation. The pathologist will send the referring physician a report stating if the biopsy was malignant or benign. Consult your physician regarding how and when you can expect to receive the biopsy results.

Infection is rare with stereotactic biopsy. However, there is a small possibility that a hematoma (a collection of blood under the skin) may develop. If this occurs, inform your physician so this information can be recorded in your medical records. This area may later show up on mammography as a change in your breast tissues.

Ultrasound

Ultrasonography, commonly referred to as an ultrasound, is a harmless test utilizing high-frequency sound waves that are sent out from a transducer, a microphone-like instrument. As the transducer moves over the breast tissue, the sound waves are bounced back to a sensor within the instrument where a picture on a monitor shows the internal structures of the breasts. These pictures, unlike a mammogram, use no radiation and allow the physician to observe the breast structures in motion. This test does not require any surgery or needles. There is no advance preparation on your part, and the test is painless.

Ultrasounds are usually used when an abnormality has been found in a breast on a mammography exam. The test determines if the suspicious area is solid tissue or a cyst filled with fluid. The ultrasound accurately locates and correctly distinguishes the makeup of a lump more than 95 percent of the time. Breast cysts are easily identified by ultrasound, which often prevents unnecessary surgery for abnormal breast lumps that cannot be felt. It is also a very useful diagnostic tool for lumps found in pregnant women, for whom mammography is not advised.

The guidance of ultrasound visualization of the lump can aid the physician in accurately locating the area for withdrawal of the fluid from a cyst or to perform a needle biopsy of the lump. Being able to see the lesion and the instrument used to withdraw fluid or perform a biopsy increases the accuracy of the procedure. Immediately following the procedure, ultrasound visualization also allows the physician to monitor the area for any changes.

There is no preparation for ultrasound. There is minimal discomfort associated with the test from the pressure of the transducer against the breast, unless it is tender, or if you cannot lie flat without discomfort. You will need to lie on a table undressed from the waist up for the test. The sonographer will apply a gel or oil substance to the breast to improve the transmission of the sound waves. The transducer will be moved over the breast while photographic images are displayed on the video monitor. A radiologist who specializes in reading ultrasound images, or sonograms, will interpret the films. The results of your ultrasound will be sent to the referring physician.

Ultrasound is not recommended by the American College of Radiology as the best method of detecting cancer by screening, but rather as an ancillary procedure after mammography has located an area that needs further evaluation. It is best used to clarify results of a mammogram or when mammography is not suitable because of pregnancy or other reasons.

Breast Cancer Genetic Testing

In 1994 and 1995, two mutated (changed) genes, BRCA1 and BRCA2 (BR=breast, CA=cancer), were discovered to cause 7 to 10 percent of breast cancers. A blood test can now determine if a person is a carrier of either of these mutated genes and the possible cause of her breast cancer. These two genes also cause a woman to be at high risk for ovarian cancer.

After a breast cancer diagnosis, the healthcare team can review your family history and personal history to determine if you meet the criteria for genetic testing. One important factor about genetic mutations is that they can be inherited from a mother or father. Breast or ovarian cancer in the history of either parent is an important consideration. For years, only the mother's family history was considered to put a woman at higher risk. We now know that the risk comes equally from the father.

Genetic testing can determine if you have a mutation in either of these genes. If positive, your children, male or female, are at a 50 percent risk of inheriting the defective genes, which they can then pass on to their offspring. Having a mutated gene places them at higher risk for breast, ovarian or other cancers.

Comparison of Cancer Risk for Normal Population and Positive Carrier

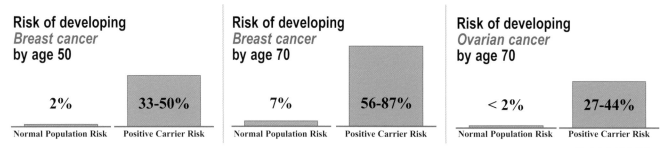

Risk of developing
Breast cancer
by age 50

2%
Normal Population Risk

33-50%
Positive Carrier Risk

Risk of developing
Breast cancer
by age 70

7%
Normal Population Risk

56-87%
Positive Carrier Risk

Risk of developing
Ovarian cancer
by age 70

< 2%
Normal Population Risk

27-44%
Positive Carrier Risk

Courtesy of Myriad Genetics

Criteria for BRCA1 or BRCA2 Testing:

- Individuals with a personal or family history of breast cancer before age 50 or ovarian cancer at any age

- Individuals with two or more primary diagnoses of breast and/or ovarian cancer

- Individuals of Ashkenazi Jewish descent with a personal or family history of breast cancer before age of 50 or ovarian cancer at any age

- Male breast cancer patients

Benefits of Testing:

- Allows one to know if their cancer was related to one of these mutated genes

- Negative test, showing no gene mutation, means that the gene for breast cancer was not passed on to children of the patient. Prevents unnecessary anxiety about children being high risk and prevents future expensive surveillance tests.

- Positive test allows family members to choose to be tested or placed in high risk surveillance programs.

- Positive test may also alter recommendations for your future treatment of breast cancer and indicate a need for surveillance for ovarian cancer or prophylactic surgical removal of your ovaries.

If you have a history of breast cancer or ovarian cancer on either side of the family, especially if breast cancer was diagnosed before menopause, discuss the benefits of genetic testing with a qualified healthcare provider. Testing consists of having a vial or syringe (several tablespoons) of blood drawn and sent to a laboratory for testing. The most appropriate person for testing is the patient with breast cancer. If you have a positive diagnosis of a mutated gene, then your offspring can be tested to see if they inherited the gene. They have approximately a 50 percent chance of inheritance. If you have a negative diagnosis, then the cause of your breast cancer is unknown and testing would not benefit your children. It is highly suggested that you be counseled about the procedure before blood is drawn and tested and after the test results are given.

Benefits of BRCA1 and BRCA2 Genetic Testing:

- Allows you to know if your breast cancer was related to one of these damaged genes.

- Allows your healthcare providers the information needed to recommend close ovarian surveillance or prophylactic oophorectomy. It also allows them to know that lumpectomy is not the recommended treatment for women who are gene carriers.

- A negative test might prevent unnecessary, expensive surveillance tests for your children.

- Allows family members to choose to be tested or placed in high-risk surveillance programs for early detection.

For up-to-date information on genetic breast cancer visit the Web site www.myriadtests.com.

UNDERSTANDING CHEMOTHERAPY DRUGS

There are many drugs used to treat breast cancer. The drugs listed below are the most common. Your physician and nursing staff will provide you with the names and side effects of the drugs you will receive.

Chemotherapy drugs are often given in combination. There are many combinations used to treat breast cancer. Often your treatment team will refer to the combination of drugs by the initials of each drug. The most common combinations are:

- CMF (Cytoxan®, Methotrexate®, 5-FU®)

- CAF (Cytoxan®, Adriamycin®, 5-FU®)

- CMFVP (Cytoxan®, Methotrexate®, 5-FU®, Vincristine®, Prednisone®)

- CFP (Cytoxan®, 5-FU®, Prednisone®)

- FAC (5-FU®, Adriamycin®, Cytoxan®)

- AC (Adriamycin®, Cytoxan®)

- ACT (Adriamycin®, Cytoxan®, Taxol® or Taxotere®)

- FEC or CEF (5-FU®, Epirubicin®, Cytoxan®)

Your treatment team may also refer to the way drugs are given by initials.

- P.O. means given by mouth.

- I.M. means given by injection into a muscle.

- S.Q. or S.C. means given by injection into the fatty (subcutaneous) tissues of the body.

- I.V. means given by a needle into a vein.

Dose Dense

Dose dense is more frequent scheduling of chemotherapy administration that shortens treatment time.

Chemotherapy Drugs

Capecitabine

Brand Name: Xeloda®

Method Administered: P.O.

Report to Physician: If pregnant, taking a blood thinner such as warfarin (Coumadin®), taking Dilatin®, the vitamin folic acid, or if you have a history of kidney or liver problems

Side Effects: Diarrhea, nausea, vomiting, stomach pain, constipation, weakness, tiredness, dizziness, headache, sleeplessness, dry or itching skin, dehydration

Notify Physician of These Side Effects: Severe diarrhea; loss of appetite; severe vomiting; tingling; numbness; pain; redness or swelling of the hands or feet; sores or pain in the mouth or throat; fever or infection; chills; sore throat; chest pain; rash

Precautions: Take drug within 30 minutes of a meal. Use barrier type method of birth control. Do not breastfeed while taking capecitabine.

Cyclophosphamide

Brand Names: Cytoxan® and Neosar®

Methods Administered: P.O., I.V.

Side Effects: Lowered blood counts (WBCs, Platelets, RBCs); nausea; vomiting; loss of appetite; hair loss; stopping menstrual periods; darkening of skin

Notify Physician of These Side Effects: Blood in urine; fever; chills; painful urination, or unusual bleeding or bruising

Precautions: Drink lots of fluids while taking medication. One to two quarts a day is recommended during the 24-hour period following administration. If the drug is given by mouth, take in the morning and follow with adequate fluids during the day.

Docetaxel

Brand Name: Taxotere®

Method Administered: I.V.

Side Effects: Temporary hair loss; decreased white blood cell count with increased risk of infection; decreased platelet count with increased risk of bleeding; hair thinning or loss; diarrhea; loss of appetite; nausea; vomiting; rash; numbness and tingling in hands or feet

Notify Physician of These Side Effects: Redness; swelling and pain in hands or feet. Contact your physician if you develop swelling in the ankles; shortness of breath; weight gain; or your clothes feel too tight at the waist.

Precautions: Some drugs increase toxicity. Consult your physician or pharmacist. Take dexamethasone (Decadron®) medication, as ordered by your physician, prior to chemotherapy.

Doxorubicin

Brand Names: Adriamycin PFS®, Adriamycin RDF®, ADR®

Method Administered: I.V.

Side Effects: Hair loss; sore mouth; nausea; vomiting; lowered blood counts (WBCs, Platelets); changes in heart rhythm; darkening of nail beds; red urine; painful urination; flu-like symptoms; sensitivity to sun or inflammation of eyes

Notify Physician of These Side Effects: Fast or irregular heartbeat; fever; chills; redness or pain at injection site; shortness of breath; swelling of feet and lower legs; diarrhea for over 24 hours; unusual bleeding or bruising; wheezing; joint pain; side or stomach pain; skin rash or itching; sores in mouth

Precautions: Causes urine to turn reddish in color hours after administration, which may stain clothing. This is not blood and will last for one to two days after administration. When the drug is being administered, if burning or pain occurs at I.V. site or in nearby veins, notify your nurse immediately. If drug leaks into tissues, necrosis will occur in area of infiltration.

Epirubicin

Brand Names: Ellence®, Pharmorubicin PFS®

Method Administered: I.V.

Side Effects: Lack of menstrual periods; nausea and vomiting; diarrhea; hot flashes; darkening of soles; palms; or nails; loss of appetite or weight loss; low white blood counts; hair loss; red urine; sore mouth

Notify Physician of These Side Effects: Severe vomiting; dehydration; fever; evidence of infection; shortness of breath; injection site pain; fast or irregular heartbeat; chills; redness or shortness of breath; swelling of feet and lower legs; diarrhea for over 24 hours; unusual bleeding or bruising; wheezing; joint pain; side or stomach pain; skin rash or itching; sores in mouth

Precautions: Tell your physician if you are taking cimetidine (Tagamet®)

Fluorouracil

Brand Names: Adrucil and 5-FU

Method Administered: I.V.

Side Effects: Lowered blood counts (WBCs, Platelets); sore mouth; nausea; vomiting; diarrhea; loss of appetite; some hair loss; sore throat; sensitivity to sunlight; darkening of skin; nail changes; dermatitis or rash; dark veins where drug was administered

Notify Physician of These Side Effects: Chest pain; cough; difficulty with balance; shortness of breath; black tarry stools; diarrhea over 24 hours in duration; fever; chills; sores in mouth; stomach cramps; unusual bleeding or bruising

Precautions: Avoid people with colds and infections. Avoid prolonged exposure to sunlight.

Gemcitabine

Brand Name: Gemzar®

Method Administered: I.V.

Side Effects: Nausea; vomiting; fatigue; diarrhea; sores in mouth or lips; flu-like symptoms with first treatment; skin rash; swelling in hands, ankles or face; thinning hair; itching

Precautions: Do not take aspirin or medicines containing aspirin.

Methotrexate

Brand Name: Folex PFS®

Methods Administered: P.O., I.M., I.V.

Side Effects: Sore mouth; nausea; vomiting; loss of appetite; diarrhea; hair loss; taste alterations; blurred vision; dizziness; fatigue; infertility; itching; sensitivity to sun

Notify Physician of These Side Effects: Black tarry stools; bloody vomit; diarrhea over 24 hours in duration; fever; chills; sore throat; sores in mouth; stomach pain, or unusual bleeding or bruising

Precautions: Do not drink alcohol while receiving the drug. Avoid too much sun and use of sun lamps or tanning beds. Do not take aspirin or ibuprofen without first checking with your physician.

Paclitaxel

Brand Name: Taxol®

Method of Administration: I.V.

Administration Side Effects: Rare allergic reaction during administration. Nurse will monitor blood pressure, temperature and respirations during infusion. **Report immediately:** shortness of breath; wheezing; dizziness or light-headedness; sudden onset of nausea; constricted feeling in throat; increase or decrease in heart rate or pain at injection site.

Expected side effects: Hair loss (occurs from 14 to 21 days after first treatment and includes: scalp, eyebrows, eyelashes and pubic hair). Lowered white blood cells. Muscle and joint pain several days after treatment. Tingling or burning sensation in hands and/or feet

Notify Physician of These Side Effects Immediately: Pain; redness or swelling at the injection site while receiving or after the drug has been given. temperature over 100.5°F; chills; blood in urine, stool, vomit or a nosebleed not controlled in 15 minutes; shortness of breath or wheezing.

Side effects that should be reported within 24 hours: Vomiting or diarrhea not controlled in 24 hours. sore throat; blisters on mouth; sores in mouth; painful or frequent urination; dizziness; any sore that does not heal or that has signs of infection (pus, redness, swelling)

Trastuzumab

Brand Name: Herceptin®

Method Administered: I.V.

Side Effects: Chills; nausea; vomiting; pain at tumor site or in abdomen or back; shortness of breath; muscle weakness or stiffness; rash; headache

Notify Physician of These Side Effects: Difficulty breathing; nausea; vomiting; diarrhea; loss of appetite; sleeplessness; unusual bruising or bleeding; swelling of the feet or ankles; rapid heartbeat; upper respiratory tract infection; excessive coughing; fever

Vincristine

Brand Names: Oncovin® and Vincasar PFS®

Method Administered: I.V.

Side Effects: Hair loss; numbness in limbs; nausea; vomiting; lowered blood counts (WBCs and platelets); ovary suppression; constipation

Notify Physician of These Side Effects: Fever; chills; unusual bleeding or bruising; blurred or double vision; confusion; constipation; difficulty walking; tingling in fingers and toes; sores in mouth; pain in stomach

Precautions: This medication can cause severe constipation. Eat lots of fiber, drink lots of water, and ask your physician about using a stool softener or laxative.

Vinorelbine

Brand Name: Navelbine®

Method Administered: I.V.

Side Effects: Redness and tenderness at site of injection; darkening of vein used; hair loss; nausea; vomiting

Notify Physician of These Side Effects: Difficulty walking; cramping in legs; redness and pain at site of I.V.; unusual bleeding or bruising; black tarry stools; lower back or side pain; fever; chills; painful or difficult urination

Precautions: Avoid people with infections.

Hormonal Drugs

Anastrazole

Brand Name: Arimidex®

Method Administered: P.O.

Side Effects: Weakness; fatigue; headache; nausea; mild diarrhea; increased or decreased appetite; sweating; hot flashes; vaginal dryness

Notify Physician of These Side Effects: Pain in lower leg; redness or swelling of your arm or leg; shortness of breath; chest pain

Exemestane

Brand Name: Aromasin®

Method Administered: P.O.

Side Effects: Fatigue; hot flashes; pain at tumor site; nausea; depression; difficulty sleeping; increased appetite; weight gain; increased sweating

Notify Physician of These Side Effects: Severe hot flashes; difficulty sleeping; depression

Precautions: Keep taking the drug even though you are feeling well. Take drug after eating.

Fulvestrant

Brand Name: Faslodex®

Method Administered: I.M.

Side Effects: Nausea; feeling listless or tired; vomiting; constipation; diarrhea; abdominal pain; headache; back pain; hot flashes; sore throat; pain at injection site; flu-like syndrome; pain in chest or pelvis

Notify Physician of These Side Effects: Bloating or swelling of face; hands; legs and feet; tingling in hands or feet; unusual weight gain or loss

Precautions: Notify physician if taking blood thinners such as Coumadin®.

Goserelin

Brand Name: Zoladex®

Method Administered: S.Q. Injection

Side Effects: Light; irregular vaginal bleeding; stopping of menstrual periods; hot flashes; headaches

Notify Physician of These Side Effects: Pelvic pain; burning; itching or dryness of vagina; anxiety; deepening of voice; increased hair growth; mental depression; mood changes; nervousness; fast or irregular heartbeat

Precautions: When taking goserelin, your menstrual period may become irregular or cease altogether. You still need to use non-hormonal birth control methods, like condoms or spermicides, if you are sexually active. Drinking alcohol while on goserelin increases risk of osteoporosis.

Letrozole

Brand Name: Femara®

Method Administered: P.O.

Side Effects: Back, bone; joint or muscle pain; hot flashes; loss of hair; weight loss; decreased appetite; sleepiness; anxiety; constipation; diarrhea; stomach pain; weakness

Notify Physician of These Side Effects: Shortness of breath; chest pain; increased sweating; severe nervousness; cough; light-headedness; sudden headache; slurred speech; sudden loss of coordination; swelling of hands or feet; vaginal bleeding

Leuprolide

Brand Names: Lupron®, Lupron Depot®, Viadur®, Leuprorelin®

Method Administered: I.M. Injection

Side Effects: Light, irregular vaginal bleeding; stopping of menstrual periods; hot flashes; blurred vision; headache; nausea or vomiting; swelling of hands or feet; swelling and tenderness of breasts; trouble sleeping; weight gain; bleeding; bruising; burning; or itching of injection site

Notify Physician of These Side Effects: Fast or irregular heartbeat; trouble breathing; sudden; severe drop in blood pressure; swelling around the eyes; rash, hives or itching; numbness or tingling in hands or feet; anxiety; deepening of voice; increased hair growth; mental depression; mood changes; nervousness

Precautions: When taking leuprorelin, your menstrual period may become irregular or cease altogether. You still need to use non-hormonal birth control methods, like condoms or spermicides, if you are sexually active.

Tamoxifen

Brand Names: Nolvadex®, TAM®

Method of Administration: P.O.

Side Effects: Hot flashes; nausea when first begun; fluid retention; vaginal discharge; menstrual irregularities; vaginal dryness; may have flare of bone pain when drug is first started (first few weeks of treatment); increase in fertility

Notify Physician of These Side Effects: Excessive vaginal dryness, vaginal infection, changes in vision, continued bone pain

Precautions: Take medication with food. Ask your physician about the need for birth control. A yearly gynecological exam is recommended.

Toremifene

Brand Name: Fareston®

Method Administered: P.O.

Side Effects: Nausea or vomiting; hot flashes; bone pain; dizziness; dry eyes

Notify Physician of These Side Effects: Blurred vision or changes in vision; change in vaginal discharge; confusion; increased urination; loss of appetite; pelvic pressure or pain; unusual tiredness; vaginal bleeding

Precautions: Taking a thiazide diuretic will increase side effects of drug. Taking Coumadin® increases risk of bleeding while on toremifene.

Miscellaneous Drugs

Dexamethasone

Brand Names: Decadron®, Dexasone®, Dexone®, Hexadrol®

Methods of Administration: P.O., I.M., I.V.

Side Effects: Euphoria; restlessness; insomnia; stomach irritation; increased appetite

Notify Physician of These Side Effects: Dizziness; fainting; shortness of breath; fever; wounds that don't heal; swelling of feet or legs

Precautions: Take medication with food. Do not take more medication than prescribed. Do not stop taking medication without informing your physician.

Dolasetron

Brand Name: Anzemet®

Method Administered: I.V. Injection, P.O.

Side Effects: Diarrhea; abdominal or stomach pain; headache; dizziness, light-headedness; fever or chills; fatigue

Notify Physician of These Side Effects: High or low blood pressure; blood in urine; painful urination; chest pain; fast heartbeat; severe stomach pain; rash, hives or itching; swelling of face, feet or lower legs; trouble breathing

Dronabinol

Brand Name: Marinol®

Method Administered: P.O.

Side Effects: Dizziness; drowsiness; nausea or vomiting; false sense of well being; trouble thinking

Notify Physician of These Side Effects (may be signs of an overdose): Amnesia; memory loss; confusion; hallucinations; delusions; anxiety; mental depression; fast heartbeat; severe drowsiness; false sense of well being; decrease in motor coordination; slurred speech; constipation; problems urinating

Precautions: Avoid alcohol and central nervous system depressants (alcohol, pain medications, tranquilizers or sleeping medication) while taking dronabinol.

Epoetin

Brand Names: Epogen®, Procrit®, Eprex®

Method Administered: Injection

Side Effects: Tiredness and weakness; tingling, burning or prickling sensation; loss of strength or energy; muscle pain

Notify Physician of These Side Effects: Chest pain; shortness of breath; seizures; coughing; sneezing; sore throat; fever; weight gain; swelling of legs, arms, feet or hands

Precautions: Epoetin may cause seizures, especially during the first 90 days of treatment; avoid driving, operating heavy machinery, and any other activities that may pose danger if a seizure occurred while you performed them.

Filgrastim

Brand Names: Neupogen®, Leukine®

Method Administered: S.Q.

Side Effects: Rash or itching; headache; pain in arms, legs, joints, muscles, lower back or pelvis

Notify Physician of These Side Effects: Redness or pain at injection site; fever; rapid or irregular heartbeat; sores on skin; wheezing

Granisetron

Brand Name: Kytril®

Method Administered: I.V., P.O.

Side Effects: Abdominal pain; constipation; diarrhea; headache; agitation; dizziness; drowsiness; heartburn; indigestion; trouble sleeping

Notify Physician of These Side Effects: Fever; severe nausea or vomiting; chest pain; fainting; irregular heartbeat; shortness of breath; rash, hives, or itching

Ondansetron

Brand Names: Zofran®, Zofran ODT®

Method Administered: I.V., P.O.

Side Effects: Constipation; diarrhea; fever; headache; abdominal pain; burning, prickling or tingling sensation; drowsiness; dry mouth; feeling cold; itching

Notify Physician of These Side Effects: Chest pain; burning, pain or redness at injection site; shortness of breath; rash, hives or itching; trouble breathing; wheezing

Oprelvelkin

Brand Name: Neumega®

Method Administered: S.Q. Injection

Side Effects: Red eyes; weakness; numbness or tingling of hands or feet; skin discoloration; rash at injection site

Notify Physician of These Side Effects: Fast or irregular heartbeat; sore mouth or tongue; white patches on mouth or tongue; shortness of breath; swelling of feet or lower legs; bloody eye; blurred vision; severe redness or peeling of skin

Pamidronate

Brand Name: Aredia®

Method Administered: I.V.

Side Effects: Abdominal pain; acid or sour stomach; belching; bladder pain; bloody or cloudy urine; body aches or pain; bone pain; cracks in skin at the corners of mouth; constipation; degenerative disease of the joint; diarrhea; difficult, burning, or painful urination; difficult or labored breathing; difficulty in moving; ear congestion; fear; frequent urge to urinate; general feeling of body discomfort or illness; heartburn; indigestion; joint pain; lack or loss of strength; loss of voice; lower back or side pain; muscle aching or cramping; muscle pains or stiffness; nasal congestion; nervousness; pain and swelling at place of injection; pain or tenderness around eyes and cheekbones; runny nose; sensitivity to heat; shivering; skin rash; sleeplessness; small clicking, bubbling, or rattling sounds in the lung when listening with a stethoscope; sneezing; soreness or redness around fingernails and toenails; stomach discomfort, upset or pain; stuffy nose; sweating; swollen joints; trouble sleeping; ulcers, sores, or white spots in mouth; unable to sleep; weight loss

Notify Physician of These Side Effects: Abdominal cramps; black, tarry stools; bleeding gums; blood in urine or stools; blurred vision; chest pain; chills; confusion; convulsions (seizures); decrease in amount of urine; dizziness; drowsiness; dry mouth; fainting; fast or irregular heartbeat; fever; headache; increased thirst; loss of appetite; mood or mental changes; muscle pain or cramps; muscle spasms; muscle twitching; nausea; nervousness; noisy, rattling breathing; numbness or tingling in hands, feet, or lips; pinpoint red spots on skin; pounding in the ears; shortness of breath; slow or fast heartbeat; sore throat; swelling of fingers, hands, feet, or lower legs; trembling; troubled breathing at rest; unusual bleeding or bruising; unusual tiredness or weakness; vomiting; vomiting of blood or material that looks like coffee grounds; weight gain

Prednisone

Brand Names: Deltasone®, Liquid Pred®, Meticorten®, Orasone®, Panasol® and Prednicen-M®.

Method Administered: P.O.

Side Effects: Increase in appetite; indigestion; nervousness; restlessness; trouble in sleeping; sense of well-being; nausea; vomiting; fluid retention

Notify Physician of These Side Effects: Blurred vision; frequent urination; hallucinations; hives or skin rash; abdominal pain or burning; black tarry stools; irregular heart beats; unusual bruising; wounds that do not heal; nausea or vomiting over 24 hours in duration

Precautions: Take medication at same time of day starting early in morning. Do not take at night or late in afternoon. Do not increase or decrease dose without physician's consent. Do not stop taking medication without notifying your physician.

RESOURCES

"As survivors, we find people who will help—friends, family, peers, support groups, role models, professional helpers, neighbors, authors, treatment programs, wig or prostheses makers—all who give good advice of various and sundry sorts to make our journey a little easier."

One of the most important ways to gain control over your disease and reduce your anxiety is to get answers to your questions. Because you are an individual, your questions and needs may be different from other women's and not addressed by your healthcare team. This is when you can reach out to support resources and find out what you need to know. The good news is that most are available free of charge. Start a notebook for keeping information about your disease, treatment and recovery. Remove the tear-out pages in the back of this book and place them in your notebook. Write down your questions and then read through this list of resources for breast cancer patients. Call or write the resource. In your notebook record your questions, the telephone number, when you called, and who you talked to. Ask them to mail you information and file it in your recovery notebook for future reference. Medication side effects information is available from your local pharmacist. Ask your healthcare team for the names of local sources of support or call your local hospital's library.

Finding Information on the Internet

The Internet is a valuable resource, but be sure that the sites you visit are recognized as having sound clinical information. Most national cancer organizations have sites, as well as medical schools and universities. Internet access is available at most public and hospital libraries if you do not have a home computer with access. Here are some suggestions for the wisest use of the Internet.

- Never substitute information found on the Internet for seeing or asking your healthcare provider about your concerns.

- Always seek information from reliable organizations and make sure that the information is dedicated to cancer education.

- Make sure the information is current. Look for the last update of the information on the site.

General Resources

AMC Cancer Research Center's Cancer Information Line
1-800-525-3777

Professional cancer counselors provide answers to questions about cancer, support and information on free publications. Equipped for deaf and hearing-impaired callers.

American Cancer Society (ACS)
www.cancer.org
1-800-ACS-2345 (1-800-227-2345)

Provides free, written information on breast cancer, support group information and referral to *Reach to Recovery* program.

Association of Cancer Online Resources
www.acor.org

Online cancer information system that archives online support groups, information on treatments and clinical trials, links to other cancer education and advocacy groups on the Internet, and much more.

BreastCancer.net
www.breastcancer.net

Archives the latest news on breast cancer and allows quick and specific searches.

BreastCancer.org
www.breastcancer.org

Breast cancer education site including articles, news, newsletter, and chats.

CancerIndex.org
www.cancerindex.org

Online index of cancer resources and Web sites providing information and support. Provides a collection of media clips on various breast cancers. To access media clips, choose "Breast Cancer" on the list on the main screen, and then click on "Multimedia Breast Cancer Resources."

Cancerlinks.org
www.cancerlinks.org

A directory of other sites and resources on specific cancers.

MEDLINEplus: Breast Cancer
www.nlm.nih.gov

Breast cancer news, general information, clinical trials and information available in Spanish.

National Cancer Institute (NCI)
www.cancer.gov
1-800-4-CANCER (1-800-422-6237)

Provides free, written information on all aspects of breast cancer.

Organizations/Advocacy Groups

Avon Breast Crusade
www.avoncrusade.com

A fundraising effort that has raised over $350 million for breast cancer education and research in countries around the world.

African-American Breast Cacner Alliance (AABCA)
www.geocities.com/aabcainc
800-ACS-2345

This organization provides education to African-American women on breast health, early detection, and breast cancer support groups. For more information and to see if there is an alliance in your area, call the American Cancer Society at 800-ACS-2345.

Cancer Care, Inc.
www.cancercare.org
1-800-813-HOPE (1-800-813-4673)

Offers free assistance to cancer patients through counseling, education, referral and direct financial assistance.

Susan G. Komen Breast Cancer Foundation
www.komen.org
1-800-IM-AWARE (1-800-462-9273)

Offers information on all areas of breast cancer treatment and support.

Native American Women and Breast Cancer
www.komen.org
1-800-IM-AWARE (1-800-462-9273)

Information on the relatively high mortality rate associated with the disease in Native American women.

National Asian Women's Heath Organization (NAWHO)
www.nawho.org

The site explains the organization's program, Communicating Across Boundaries: The Asian American Woman's Breast and Cervical Cancer Program, and offers a free download on related cultural competency training.

National Breast Cancer Coalition
www.natlbcc.org
1-202-296-7477

A grassroots advocacy movement of more than 300 member organizations and thousands of individuals working through a National Action Network, dedicated to the eradication of breast cancer through action, policy and advocacy.

Y-ME National Breast Cancer Organization
www.y-me.org
1-800-221-2141 (24 Hour Hotline-English)
1-800-986-9505 (24 Hour Hotline-Spanish)

Provides support and counseling through a 24-hour hotline. Trained volunteers, all of whom have had breast cancer, are matched by background and experience to callers whenever possible. Referrals for major cancer treatment centers available.

The Young Survival Coalition
www.youngsurvival.org
1-212-206-6610

An advocacy and awareness organization for young women who are diagnosed with breast cancer. The group offers support, information and education.

Breast Reconstruction

American Cancer Society

Breast Reconstruction after Mastectomy

www.cancer.org (in search box on home page type in "breast reconstruction")

A thorough explanation of reconstruction options and goals for the mastectomy patient.

Breast Implants

Food and Drug Administration Breast Implant Information

www.fda.gov

Call 1-888-463-6332

Information on choosing an implant, the associated risks, FDA regulations, and manufacturers of implants.

Cancer Treatment

www.cancer.gov

The National Cancer Institute maintains a cancer treatment database providing prognostic, stage and treatment information on more than 1,000 protocol (treatment) summaries.

National Comprehensive Cancer Network: Breast Cancer Treatment Guidelines for Patients

www.nccn.org

Decision trees included in this site aid patients in choosing treatment and follow-up options. Also available in Spanish.

Children

Kids Konnected

www.kidskonnected.org

1-800-899-2866

Kids Konnected is a non-profit organization that provides for the needs of the children of cancer patients. They offer a kid-friendly and informative Web site, a 24-hour hotline, leadership training, support groups, online forums, a teddy bear outreach program, and other support tools for children and families.

Clinical Aspects

Cancer.gov: Breast Cancer Clinical Trials

www.cancer.gov/clinicaltrials/

Information on choosing and participating in clinical trials, results of recent trials, and resources for finding a trial.

Inflammatory Breast Cancer (IBC) Research Foundation

www.ibcresearch.org

General information, research, articles, news articles, discussion and commentary on inflammatory breast cancer.

Hair Care and Make-Up

Look Good, Feel Better

www.lookgoodfeelbetter.org

1-800-395-LOOK (5665)

Call your local ACS office. A program of the American Cancer Society that offers free class instructions on makeup application and hair care during cancer treatment.

Male Breast Cancer

ACS: Male Breast Cancer Resource Center

www.cancer.org (in search box on home page type in "male breast cancer")

Information and other Web sites on male breast cancer.

Pregnancy and Breast Cancer

Fertile Hope

www.fertilehope.org

Fertile Hope is a national non-profit organization dedicated to providing reproductive information, support and hope to cancer patients whose medical treatments present the risk of infertility.

Pregnant With Cancer Network

www.pregnantwithcancer.org
1-800-743-4471

Connects pregnant women diagnosed with cancer to women who have lived through the experience.

Prosthesis

Check in the yellow pages of your telephone book. Call your local unit of the American Cancer Society. Ask your surgeon or nurse for references.

Y-ME

www.y-me.org
800-221-2141 (English)/800-986-9505 (Spanish)

This organization maintains a prosthesis and wig bank for women who cannot afford to purchase one. If the appropriate size of prosthesis or color of wig is available, it will be mailed anywhere in the country to you for a small shipping fee.

Support Groups

Call your local **American Cancer Society** office or National office at 800-ACS-2345.

Y-ME at 800-221-2141.

Survivorship Magazines

Coping with Cancer

www.copingmag.com
615-790-2400

Coping With Cancer is America's consumer magazine for people whose lives have been touched by cancer. This magazine provides knowledge, hope, and inspiration to cancer patients, survivors and their families. For a subscription go online or call.

CURE

www.curetoday.com
800-210-CURE (2873)

CURE is a magazine for cancer patients and their families, providing information on recent advancements in diagnosis, treatment and prevention of cancer. Healthcare providers and patients can go online to sign up for a free subscription.

MAMM

www.mamm.com
646-365-1350

MAMM is a magazine devoted to women diagnosed with breast and reproductive cancer. It helps women to understand more about their diagnosis, improve the quality of their life and assess current treatments as well as new therapies on the horizon. For a subscription go online or call.

Survivorship Resources

Imaginis
www.imaginis.com

Excellent web site for professionals and patients providing education and the latest news in breast cancer. Sign up for the online newsletter to receive concise summaries on the latest news and information on breast cancer.

Living Beyond Breast Cancer (LBBC)
www.lbbc.org
Phone: 610-645-4567 Fax: 610-645-4573
10 East Athens Ave. Suite 204
Ardmore, PA 19903

LBBC is a non-profit educational organization committed to empowering all women affected by breast cancer to live as long as possible with the best quality of life. Programs include semi-annual large scale educational conferences, a quarterly newsletter, educational teleconferencing programs, outreach to medically underserved women, and a consumer focused educational booklet.

Living With It
www.livingwithit.org

"Living with it" is a program created by Aventis Oncology for women with breast cancer. It is a web and mail based program providing patients with survivor stories, diet and exercise tips, medical information, treatment organizers, and other valuable information. Patients can go online to sign up.

National Coalition for Cancer Survivorship (NCCS)
www.canceradvocacy.org
1-877-NCCS-YES (877-622-7937)

Survivorship information and support. Cancer Survival Toolbox, a CD of Survival Skills, provided free (available in Spanish).

Patient Advocate Foundation (Employment Issues)
www.patientadvocate.org
800-532-5274

The Patient Advocate Foundation is a national non-profit organization that serves as an active liaison between the patient and her insurer, employer and/or debt crisis matters relative to their diagnosis through case managers, doctors and attorneys. Patient Advocate Foundation seeks to safeguard patients through effective mediation assuring access to care, maintenance of employment and preservation of their financial stability.

Reach To Recovery
National ACS Office 800-ACS-2345

A program of the American Cancer Society, offers visits from volunteers. Call your local ACS unit for an appointment. Volunteers will share helpful information for recovery, including range of motion exercises for the surgical arm.

The Wellness Community
www.thewellnesscommunity.org
Phone: 202-659-9709 Fax: 202-659-9301
919 18th Street NW Suite 54
Washington, DC 20006

The Wellness Community is a national non-profit organization dedicated to providing free emotional support, education and hope for people with cancer. There are 20 facilities nationwide. The web offers online support groups and an online newsletter for cancer patients.

RECOMMENDED READING

Breast Cancer Survivors' Club:
A Nurse's Experience
Lillie Shockney
Publisher: Real Health Books
ISBN: 0970460104
April, 2001

The Human Side of Cancer:
Living with Hope, Coping with Uncertainty
Jimmie C. Holland, MD
Sheldon Lewis
Publisher: Harper Collins Publishers
ISBN: 006093042X
October, 2001

Life Strategies: Doing What Works,
Doing What Matters
Phillip C. McGraw, Ph.D.
Publisher: Hyperion
ISBN: 0641640617
January, 2000

Timeless Healing
Herbert Benson, Mark Stark
Publisher: Simon & Schuster Adult Publishing Group
ISBN: 0684831465
March, 1997

Sexuality and Fertility after Cancer
Leslie R. Schover
Publisher: Wiley, John &Sons, Inc.
ISBN: 0471181943
September, 1997

Eating Well, Staying Well:
During and After Cancer
Abby Bloch, Ph.D.
Michelle D. Cassileth, M.D.
Cynthia A. Thomson, Ph.D.
Publisher: American Cancer Society
ISBN: 0944235514
July, 2004

Helping Your Mate Face Breast Cancer
Tips for Becoming An Effective Support Partner
Judy C. Kneece, RN, OCN
Publisher: EduCare Inc.
ISBN: 1886665117
June, 2003

Talking With Kids About Cancer
Dave Dravecky, Outreach of Hope
1-719-481-3528
outreachofhope.org

REFERENCES

American Joint Committee on Cancer Staging Manual, 6th Edition
Frederick L. Greene, MD
David L. Page, MD
Irvin D. Fleming, MD
April G. Fritz, C.T.R., R.H.I.T.
Charles M. Balch, MD
Daniel G. Haller, MD
Monica Morrow, MD
Springer-Verlag 2002

The Breast: Comprehensive Management of Benign and Malignant Diseases
Kirby I. Bland, MD
Edward Copeland, III, MD
W. B. Saunders Company
Philadelphia 1998

Clinical Oncology
Raymond E. Lenhard, Jr. MD
Robert T. Osteen MD
Ted Gansler MD
American Cancer Society
Blackwell Publishers
2001

Diseases of the Breast
Jay R. Harris
Marc E. Lippman, MD
Monica Morrow, MD
Kent C. Osborne, MD
Lippincott Williams & Wilkins
Philadelphia 2004

Lippincott's Nursing Drug Guide, 2004
Amy M. Karch
Springhouse Publishing
Philadelphia 2003

MammaCare® Method of Breast Self-Exam
Gainesville, Florida
MammaTech Corp
H. S. Pennypacker
www.mammacare.com

Psycho-Oncology
Jimmie C. Holland, MD
William Breitbart
Oxford University Press 1998

Surgery of the Breast: Principles and Art
Scott L. Spear, MD
John W. Little. MD
Marc E. Lippman, MD
William C. Wood, MD
Philadelphia, Lippincott Williams & Wilkins 1998

GLOSSARY

It is important to understand the medical terminology related to your diagnosis and treatments. The following is a list of the most common medical terms used in breast cancer. If you do not understand the technical language used by your doctor or nurse, ask them to explain what they mean. Understanding the terms will enable you to make intelligent decisions.

A

Abscess — A collection of pus from infection.

Acini — The parts of the breast gland where fluid or milk is produced (singular: acinus).

Acute — Occurring suddenly or over a short period of time.

Adenocarcinoma — A form of cancer that involves cells from the lining of the walls of many different organs of the body. Breast cancer is a type of adenocarcinoma.

Adjuvant Treatment — Treatment that is added to increase the effectiveness of a primary treatment. In cancer, adjuvant treatment usually refers to chemotherapy, hormonal therapy or radiation therapy after surgery to increase the likelihood of killing all cancer cells.

Alkylating Agent — Type of chemotherapy drug used in cancer treatment.

Alopecia — Refers to hair loss as a result of chemotherapy or radiation therapy administered to the head. Hair loss from chemotherapy is temporary. Hair loss from radiation is usually permanent.

Amenorrhea — The absence or discontinuation of menstrual periods.

Analgesic — Medicine given to control pain; for example: Aspirin or Tylenol®.

Anesthesia — Medication that causes entire or partial loss of feeling or sensation.

ASK QUESTIONS.

BE INFORMED.

LIVE ONE DAY AT A TIME.

— JUDY M. SHEEKS
Survivor

Androgen — A male sex hormone. Androgens may be used in patients with breast cancer to treat recurrence of the disease.

Aneuploid — The characteristic of having either fewer or more than the normal number of chromosomes in a cell. This is an abnormal cell.

Anorexia — Severe, uncontrolled loss of appetite.

Antiemetic — A medicine that prevents or relieves nausea and vomiting; used during and sometimes after chemotherapy.

Antimetabolites — Anticancer drugs that interfere with the process of DNA production, thus preventing cell division.

Areola — The circular field of dark colored skin surrounding the nipple.

Aspiration — Removal of fluid or cells from tissue by inserting a needle into an area and drawing the fluid into the syringe.

Asymptomatic — Without obvious signs or symptoms of disease. While cancer may cause symptoms and warning signs, it may develop and grow without producing any symptoms, especially in its early stages.

Atypical Cells — Not usual; abnormal. Cancer is the result of atypical cell division.

Axilla — The armpit.

Axillary Dissection — Surgical removal of lymph nodes from the armpit. The tissue removed is sent to the pathologist to determine if the breast cancer has spread outside of the breast. The number of nodes dissected varies during surgery. Your physician can tell you how many nodes were removed.

Axillary Nodes — The lymph nodes in the axilla (underarm). These nodes may be cut out and examined during surgery to see if the cancer has spread past the breast. The number of nodes in this area varies.

ABSOLUTELY NOTHING

IN MY LIFE PREPARED

ME FOR CANCER—

EXCEPT GOD.

—KAY C. HARVEY
Survivor

B

Benign Tumor — An abnormal growth that is not cancer and does not spread to other parts of the body.

Bilateral — Pertains to both sides of the body. For example, bilateral breast cancer would be on both sides of the body or in two breasts.

Biological Response Modifier — Treatment used that alters the body's natural response to stimulate bone marrow to make specific blood cells. Referred to as a colony stimulating factor.

Biopsy — The surgical removal of a small piece of tissue or a small tumor for microscopic examination to determine if cancer cells are present. A biopsy is the most important procedure in diagnosing cancer.

Biotherapy — Treatments used to stimulate the body's immune system.

Blood Count — A test to measure the number of red blood cells (RBCs), white blood cells (WBCs) and platelets in a blood sample.

Bone Marrow — The soft, fatty substance filling the cavities of the bones. Blood cells are manufactured in the bone marrow. Chemotherapy affects the bone marrow, resulting in a temporary decrease in the number of cells in the blood.

Bone Marrow Biopsy and Aspiration — A procedure in which a needle is inserted into the center of a bone, usually the hip, to remove a small amount of bone marrow for microscopic examination.

Bone Scan — A procedure in which a trace amount of radioactive substance is injected into the bloodstream to illuminate the bones under a special camera to see if the cancer has spread to the bones.

Breast Cancer — A potentially fatal tumor, because of its ability to leave the breast and go to other vital organs and continue to grow if it is not removed from the body. These are uncontrolled breast cells that are abnormal with uncontrolled growth.

Breast Implant — A round or teardrop shaped sac inserted into the body to restore the shape of the breast. May be filled with saline water or synthetic material.

Breast Self-Exam (BSE) — A procedure to examine the breasts thoroughly once a month to detect any changes or suspicious lumps. Exams should be practiced at the end of the menstrual period or seven days after the start of the period and should be performed monthly at the same time.

BREAST CANCER PROMPTS

A DESIRE TO TAKE ACTION.

—*JUDY E. WINDSOR*
Survivor

C

Calcifications — Small calcium deposits in breast tissue seen on mammography. The smallest object detected on mammography. Deposits are the result of cell death. Occurs with benign and malignant changes.

Cancer — A general term used to describe more than 100 different uncontrolled growths of abnormal cells in the body. Cancer cells have the ability to continue to grow, invade and destroy surrounding tissue, leave the original site and travel via lymph or blood systems to other parts of the body where they can set up new cancerous tumors.

Cancer Cell — A cell that divides and reproduces abnormally with uncontrolled growth. This cell can break away and travel to other parts of the body and set up another site; this is referred to as metastasis.

Clavicle — The collarbone.

Carcinoembryonic Antigen (CEA) — A blood test used to follow women with metastatic breast cancer to help determine if the treatment is working. This is not a test specific for cancer.

Carcinogen — Any substance that initiates or promotes the development of cancer. For example, asbestos is a proven carcinogen.

Carcinoma — A form of cancer that develops in tissues covering or lining organs of the body, such as the skin, the uterus, the lung or the breast.

Carcinoma In Situ — An early stage of development, when the cancer is still confined to the tissues of origin. It has not spread outside the area. In situ carcinomas are highly curable.

CAT Scan or CT Scan — An x-ray view of the body in sections.

Cell — The basic structural unit of all life. All living matter is composed of cells.

Cellulitis — Infection occurring in soft tissues. Your surgical arm has an increased risk for cellulitis because of the removal of lymph nodes. Pain, swelling and warmth occur in the area.

Chemotherapy — Treatment of cancer by use of chemicals. Usually refers to drugs used to treat cancer.

Clinical Trial — A scientific study, generally involving a large number of test subjects (or patients), that is conducted to prove or determine the effectiveness of a drug or treatment program. Limited experimental evidence and preliminary studies prior to the clinical trial has shown or suggested the potential effectiveness and usefulness of the drug or treatment.

CANCER HAS GIVEN
ME A PURPOSE.
IT HAS MOST ASSUREDLY
OPENED BOTH MY EYES
AND MY HEART.

—*ROSE-MARIE BOWMAN GANN*
Survivor

Combination Chemotherapy — Treatment consisting of the use of two or more chemicals to achieve maximum kill of tumor cells.

Combined Modality Therapy — Two or more types of treatments used to supplement each other. For instance, surgery, radiation, chemotherapy, hormonal or immunotherapy may be used alternatively or together for maximum effectiveness.

Complete Blood Count (CBC) — A laboratory test to determine the number of red blood cells, white blood cells, platelets, hemoglobin and other components of a blood sample.

Computerized Tomography Scans — Commonly called CT or CAT scans. These specialized x-ray studies indicate cancer or metastasis.

Cooper's Ligaments — Flexible fibrous elastic bands of tissue pass from the chest muscle into the breast tissues between the lobes of the breasts, providing shape and support for the breasts.

Core Biopsy — Removal (with a large needle) of a piece of a lump. The piece is sent to the lab to see if the lump is benign or malignant.

Cyst — An abnormal sac-like structure that contains liquid or semisolid material; is usually benign. Lumps in the breast are often found to be harmless cysts.

Cytology — The study of cells under a microscope that have been sloughed off, cut out or scraped off organs; cells are microscopically examined for signs of cancer.

Cytotoxic — Drugs that can cause the death of cancer cells. Usually refers to drugs used in chemotherapy treatments.

D

Detection — The discovery of an abnormality in an asymptomatic or symptomatic person.

Diagnosis — The process of identifying a disease by its characteristic signs, symptoms and laboratory findings. With cancer, the earlier the diagnosis is made, the better the chance for a cure.

Diaphanography (DPG) — A non-invasive procedure (no cutting) that uses ordinary light as an investigative tool to detect breast masses. Also called transillumination.

Differentiated — The similarity between a normal cell and the cancer cell; defines what degree of change has occurred. Cancer cells that are well differentiated are close to the original cell and are usually less aggressive. Poorly differentiated cells have changed more and are more aggressive.

CRY WHEN YOU MUST. REMEMBER, IT COULD BE WORSE. JUST DO YOUR BEST. CRY AND YOU'LL FEEL BETTER. DANCE ALSO IF POSSIBLE.

—*AUDREY E. MITCHELL*
Survivor

Diploid — The characteristic of having two sets of chromosomes in a cell. This is normal for a breast cell.

DNA — One of two nucleic acids (the other is RNA) found in the nucleus of all cells. DNA contains genetic information on cell growth, division and cell function.

Doubling Time — The time required for a cell to double in number. Breast cancer has been shown to double in size every 23 to 209 days. It would take one cell, doubling every 100 days, eight to ten years to reach one centimeter, 3/8 inch.

Ductal Carcinoma In Situ — A cancer inside the ducts of breast that has not grown through the wall of the duct into the surrounding tissues. Sometimes referred to as a precancer. Good prognosis is involved with in situ cancers.

Ductal Papillomas — Small noncancerous finger-like growths in the mammary ducts that may cause a bloody nipple discharge. Commonly found in women 45 to 50 years of age.

E

Edema — Excess fluid in the body or a body part that is described as swollen or puffy.

Endocrine Manipulation — Treating breast cancer by changing the hormonal balance of the body to prevent hormone dependent cancer cells from multiplying.

Estrogen — A female hormone, secreted by the ovaries, that is essential for menstruation, reproduction and the development of secondary sex characteristics, such as breasts. Some patients with breast cancer are given drugs to suppress the production of estrogen in their bodies.

Estrogen Receptor Assay (ERA) — A test that is done on cancerous tissue to see if a breast cancer is hormone-dependent and may be treated with hormonal therapy. The test will reveal if your cancer is estrogen receptor positive or negative.

Excisional Biopsy — Surgical removal of a lump or suspicious tissue by cutting the skin and removing the tissue.

F

Familial Cancer — One occurring in families more frequently than would be expected by chance.

Fat Necrosis Tumor — A hard noncancerous lump caused by the destruction of fat cells in the breast due to trauma or injury.

Fibroadenoma — A noncancerous, solid tumor most commonly found in younger women.

Fibrocystic Breast Changes or Condition — A noncancerous breast condition in which multiple cysts or lumpy areas develop in one or both breasts. It can be accompanied by discomfort or pain that fluctuates with the menstrual cycle. Large cysts can be treated by aspiration of the fluid they contain.

Fine Needle Aspiration — A procedure to remove cells or fluid from tissues using a needle with an empty syringe. Cells or breast fluid, extracted by pulling back on the plunger, are analyzed by a physician.

Flow Cytometry — A test done on cancerous tissues that shows the aggressiveness of the tumor. It shows how many cells are in the dividing stage at one time, commonly referred to as the 'S' phase, and the DNA content of the cancer, referred to as the ploidy. This reveals how rapidly the tumor is growing.

Frozen Section — A technique in which a part of the biopsy tissue is frozen immediately, and a thin slice of frozen tissue is mounted on a microscope slide for a diagnostic examination by a pathologist.

Frozen Shoulder — Surgical shoulder which has a severely restricted range of motion and is painful.

G

Galactocele — A clogged milk duct often associated with childbirth.

Genes — Segments of DNA that contain hereditary information that is transferred from cell to cell; genes are located in the nucleus of the cell.

Genetic — Refers to the inherited pattern located in genes for certain characteristics.

H

Hematoma — A collection of blood that can form in a wound after surgery, an aspiration or from an injury.

Hormonal Therapy — Treatment of cancer by alteration of the hormonal balance. Some cancer will only grow in the presence of certain hormones.

Hormones — Chemicals secreted by various organs in the body that help regulate growth, metabolism and reproduction. Some hormones are used as treatment following surgery for breast, ovarian and prostate cancers.

FINDING THE HUMOR IN BREAST CANCER HAS BROUGHT ME TREMENDOUS PHYSICAL AND PSYCHOLOGICAL HEALING.

—*JANE HILL*
Survivor

GET THE FACTS ABOUT YOUR CANCER. IT IS THE ONLY WAY YOU CAN MAKE AN INFORMED DECISION.

— *Survivor*

HUMOR HELPS.
GO OUT EACH DAY WITH JOY.

—*MILDRED HYDRICK*
Survivor

Hormone Receptor Assay — A diagnostic test to determine whether a breast cancer's growth is influenced by hormones or if it can be treated with hormones.

Hot Flashes — A sensation of heat and flushing that occurs suddenly. May be associated with menopause or some medications.

Hyperplasia — An abnormal excessive growth of cells that is benign.

I

Intramuscular (I.M.) — To receive a medication by needle injection into the muscle of the body.

Immune System — A complex system by which the body protects itself from outside invaders that are harmful to the body.

Immunology — The study of the body's mechanisms of resistance against disease and invasion by foreign substances—the body's ability to fight a disease.

Immunotherapy — A treatment that stimulates the body's own defense mechanisms to combat diseases such as cancer.

Immunosuppressed — Condition of having a lowered resistance to disease. May be a temporary result of lowered white blood cells from chemotherapy administration.

Incisional Biopsy — A surgical incision made through the skin to remove a portion of a suspected lump or tissue.

Inflammation — Reaction of tissue to various conditions that may result in pain, redness or warmth of tissues in the area.

Infiltrating Cancer — Cancer that has grown through the cell wall of the breast area in which it originated, and into the surrounding tissues.

Informed Consent — Process of explaining to the patient the risks and complications of a procedure or treatment before it is done. Most informed consents are written and signed by the patient or a legal representative.

Intraductal — Residing within the duct of the breast. Intraductal disease may be benign or malignant.

Invasive Cancer — Cancer that has spread outside its site of origin and is growing into the surrounding tissues.

In Situ — In place, localized and confined to one area. A very early stage of cancer.

INFORMATION ABOUT MY
CANCER WAS NECESSARY FOR
ME TO ONCE AGAIN FEEL
IN CONTROL OF MY LIFE.

—*ANN PARKER*
Survivor

Infiltrating Ductal Carcinoma — A cancer that begins in the mammary glands and has spread to areas outside the gland.

Intravenous (I.V.) — Entering the body through a vein.

Inverted Nipple — The turning inward of the nipple. Usually a congenital condition; but, if it occurs where it has not previously existed, it can be a sign of breast cancer.

L

Lactation — Process of being able to produce milk from the breasts.

Lesion — An area of tissue that is diseased.

Leukocyte — A white blood cell or corpuscle.

Leukopenia — A decrease in the number of white blood cells (where the count is less than 5000); increases a person's susceptibility to infection.

Linear Accelerator — A machine that produces high-energy x-ray beams to destroy cancer cells.

Liver Scan — A way of visualizing the liver by injecting into the bloodstream a trace dose of a radioactive substance which helps visualize the organ during x-ray.

Lobular — Pertaining to the part of the breast that is furthest from the nipple, the lobes.

Localized Cancer — A cancer still confined to its site of origin.

Lump — Any kind of abnormal mass in the breast or elsewhere in the body.

Lumpectomy — A surgical procedure in which only the cancerous tumor and an area of surrounding tissue is removed. Usually the surgeon will remove some of the underarm lymph nodes at the same time. This procedure is also referred to as a tylectomy.

Lymph — A clear fluid circulating throughout the body in the lymphatic system that contains white blood cells and antibodies.

Lymph Glands — Also called lymph nodes. These are rounded body tissues in the lymphatic system that vary in size from a pinhead to an olive and may appear in groups or one at a time. The principal ones are in the neck, underarm and groin. These glands produce lymphocytes and monocytes (white blood cells which fight foreign substances) and serve as filters to prevent bacteria from entering the bloodstream. They will filter out cancer cells but will also serve as a site for metastatic disease. The major ones serving the breast are in the armpit. Some are located above and below the collarbone and some in between the ribs near the

LIVE LIFE ONE DAY AT A TIME. YOU CAN'T CHANGE YESTERDAY. FORGET THOSE "IF ONLY" THOUGHTS. WORRYING ABOUT TOMORROW ONLY MAKES THINGS WORSE.

—HARRIETT BARRINEAU
  Survivor

breast-bone. There are three levels of lymph nodes in the underarm area of the breast and another around the breastbone. The number of nodes varies from person to person. Lymph nodes are usually sampled during surgery to determine if the cancer has spread outside of the breast area.

Lymphatic Vessels — Vessels that remove cellular waste from the body by filtering through lymph nodes and eventually emptying into the vascular (blood) system.

Lymphedema — A swelling in the arm (or extremities) caused by excess fluid that collects after the lymph nodes have been removed by surgery or affected by radiation treatments.

M

Macrocyst — A cyst that is large enough to be felt with the fingers.

Magnification View — Special enlarged views to magnify an area for greater detail of suspicious finding. Used in mammography.

Magnetic Resonance Imaging (MRI) — A magnet scan; a form of x-ray using magnets instead of radiation. MRI gives a more clearly defined picture of fatty tissue than x-ray.

Malignant Tumor — A mass of cancer cells. These cells have uncontrolled growth and will invade surrounding tissues and spread to distant sites of the body, setting up new cancer sites; this process is called metastasis.

Mammary Duct Ectasia — A noncancerous breast disease most often found in women during menopause. The ducts in or beneath the nipple become clogged with cellular and fatty debris. The duct may have gray to greenish discharge, a lump you can feel, and can become inflamed, causing pain.

Mammary Glands — The breast glands that produce and carry milk by way of the mammary ducts to the nipples during pregnancy and breastfeeding.

Mammogram — An x-ray of the breast that can detect tumors before they can be felt. A baseline mammogram is performed on healthy breasts usually at the age of 35 to establish a basis for later comparison.

Mammotest — Biopsy (stereotactic) performed under mammography while breast is compressed and the lesion is viewed by physician. Sample of lesion is removed using a large core needle and is then sent to the lab to determine if it is benign or malignant.

Margins — The area of tissue surrounding a tumor when it is removed by surgery.

MUSIC HAS ALWAYS BEEN AN IMPORTANT PART OF MY LIFE. WHENEVER I FELT THE NEED FOR A BOOST, I'D START SINGING.

—*LOUISE K. EDWARDS*
Survivor

Mastalgia — Pain occurring in the breast.

Mastectomy — Surgical removal of the breast and some of the surrounding tissue.

> **Modified Radical Mastectomy** — The most common type of mastectomy. Breast skin, nipple, areola and underarm lymph nodes are removed. The chest muscles are saved.

> **Prophylactic Mastectomy** — A preventative procedure sometimes recommended for patients at a very high risk for developing cancer in one or both sides.

> **Subcutaneous Mastectomy** — Performed before cancer is detected. A procedure that removes the breast tissue but leaves the outer skin, areola and nipple intact. (This is not suitable with a diagnosis of cancer.)

> **Radical Mastectomy (Halsted Radical)** — The surgical removal of the breast, breast skin, nipple, areola, chest muscles and underarm lymph nodes.

> **Segmental Mastectomy (Partial Mastectomy/Lumpectomy)** — A surgical procedure in which only a portion of the breast is removed, including the cancer and the surrounding margin of healthy breast tissue.

Mastitis — An infection occurring in the breast. Pain, tenderness, swelling, redness and warmth may be observed. Usually responds to antibiotic treatment.

Menopause — The time in a woman's life when the menstrual cycle ends and the ovaries produce lower levels of hormones; usually occurs between the age of 45 and 55.

Metastasis — The spread of cancer from one part of the body to another through the lymphatic system or the bloodstream. The cells in the new cancer location are the same type as those in the original site.

Microcalcifications — Particles observed on a mammogram that are found in the breast tissue, appearing as small spots on the picture. Usually occur from calcium deposits caused by death of breast cells that may be benign or malignant. When clustered in one area, may need to be checked more closely for a malignant change in the breast.

Microcyst — A cyst that is too small to be felt but may be observed on mammography or ultrasound screening.

Micrometastasis — The undetectable spread of cancer outside of the breast that is not seen on routine screening tests. Metastasis is too limited to have created enough mass to be observed.

MEDICAL BILLS HAVE BEEN OVERWHELMING. BUT, BY THE GRACE OF GOD, I'M TRYING.

—Survivor

Multicentric — More than one origin or place of growth in the breast. These growths may or may not be related to each other.

Myleosuppression — A decrease in the ability of the bone marrow cells to produce blood cells, including red blood cells, white blood cells and platelets. This condition increases susceptibility to infection and produces fatigue.

N

Needle Biopsy — Removal of a sample of tissue from the breast using a wide-core needle with suction.

Necrosis — Death of a tissue.

Neoplasm — Any abnormal growth. Neoplasms may be benign or malignant, but the term usually is used to describe a cancer.

Nodularity — Increased density of breast tissue, most often due to hormonal changes, which cause the breast to feel lumpy in texture. This finding is called normal nodularity, and it usually occurs in both breasts.

Nodule — A small, solid mass.

O

Oncogene — Certain stretches of cellular DNA. Genes that, when inappropriately activated, contribute to the malignant transformation of a cell.

Oncologist — A physician who specializes in cancer treatment.

Oncology — The science dealing with the physical, chemical and biological properties and features of cancer, including causes, the disease process, and therapies.

One-Step Procedure — A procedure in which a surgical biopsy is performed under general anesthesia and if cancer is found, a mastectomy or lumpectomy is done immediately as part of the same operation.

Oophorectomy — The surgical removal of the ovaries, sometimes performed as a part of hormone therapy.

Orgasm — A state of physical and emotional excitement that occurs at the climax of sexual intercourse.

Osteoporosis — Softening of bones that occurs with age, calcium loss and hormone depletion.

NOTHING IS MORE FRIGHTENING THAN THE WORD, "CANCER."

—*Survivor*

OVERCOMING FEAR IS THE FIRST STEP TO SURVIVAL.

—*LISA BOCCARD*
Survivor

P

Per Orally (P.O.) — To take a medication by mouth.

Palliative Treatment — Therapy that relieves symptoms, such as pain or pressure, but does not alter the development of the disease. Its primary purpose is to improve the quality of life.

Palpation — A procedure using the hands to examine organs such as the breast. A palpable mass is one you can feel with your hands.

Pathology — The study of disease through the microscopic examination of body tissues and organs. Any tumor suspected of being cancerous must be diagnosed by pathological examination.

Pathologist — A physician with special training in diagnosing diseases from samples of tissue.

Pectoralis Muscles — Muscular tissues attached to the front of the chest wall and extending to the upper arms. These are under the breast. They are divided into the pectoralis major and the pectoralis minor muscles.

Permanent Section — A technique in which a thin slice of biopsy tissue is mounted on a slide to be examined under a microscope by a pathologist in order to establish a diagnosis.

Platelet — A cell formed by the bone marrow and circulating in the blood that is necessary for blood clotting. Platelet transfusions are used in cancer patients to prevent or control bleeding when the number of platelets has decreased.

Ploidy — The number of chromosome sets in a cell.

Port, Life Port, Port-A-Cath — A device surgically implanted under the skin, usually on the chest, that enters a large blood vessel and is used to deliver medication, chemotherapy, blood products and also is used to obtain blood samples. A port is usually inserted if a person has veins in the arm that are difficult to use for treatment or if certain types of chemotherapy drugs are to be given.

Precancerous — Abnormal cellular changes that are potentially capable of becoming cancer. These early lesions are very amenable to treatment and cure. Also called pre-malignant.

Progesterone — Female hormone produced by the ovaries during a specific time in the menstrual cycle. Causes the uterus to prepare for pregnancy and the breasts to get ready to produce milk.

Progesterone Receptor Assay (PRA) — A test that is done on cancerous tissue to see if a breast cancer is progesterone hormone dependent and can be treated by hormonal therapy.

PEOPLE HURT.

THE HUMAN SPIRIT

IS SENSITIVE TO LOSS. THIS IS

NORMAL. EMOTIONAL HEALING

MAY TAKE LONGER THAN

YOUR PHYSICAL HEALING.

—*Survivor*

Prognosis — A prediction of the course of the disease-the future prospect for the patient. For example, most breast cancer patients who receive treatment early have a good prognosis.

Prolactin — A female hormone that stimulates the development of the breasts and later is essential for starting and continuing milk production.

Prophylactic Mastectomy — Removal of high-risk breast tissue to prevent future development of cancer.

Prosthesis — An artificial form. In the case of post-mastectomy breast cancer patients, a breast form that can be worn inside a bra.

Protocol — A schedule of selected drugs and treatment time intervals known to be effective against a certain cancer.

R

Radiation Therapy — Treatment with high energy x-rays to destroy cancer cells.

Radiation Oncologist — A physician specifically trained in the use of high energy x-rays to treat cancer.

Radiologist — A physician who specializes in diagnoses of diseases by the use of x-rays.

Radiotherapy — Treatment of cancer with high-energy radiation. Radiation therapy may be used to reduce the size of a cancer before surgery or to destroy any remaining cancer cells after surgery. Radiotherapy can be helpful in shrinking recurrent cancer to relieve symptoms such as pain and pressure.

Recurrence — Reappearance of cancer after a period of remission.

Regional Involvement — The spread of cancer from its original site to nearby surrounding areas. Regional cancers are confined to one location of the body. Regional involvement in breast cancer could include the spread to the lymph nodes or to the chest wall.

Rehabilitation — Programs that help patients adjust and return to full, productive lives. May involve physical therapy, the use of a prosthesis, counseling and emotional support.

Relapse — The reappearance of cancer after a disease-free period.

Remission — Complete or partial disappearance of the signs and symptoms of disease in response to treatment. The period during which a disease is under control. A remission, however, is not necessarily a cure.

Retraction — The process of skin pulling in toward breast tissue, often referred to as dimpling.

Risk Factors — Anything that increases an individual's chance of getting a disease such as cancer. The risk factors for breast disease include having a first degree relative with breast cancer, a high fat diet, early menstruation, late menopause, first child after 30 or no children.

Risk Reduction — Techniques used to reduce your chances of getting a certain cancer. For example, reducing your dietary fat may help prevent breast cancer.

S

S Phase — A test that is performed to determine how many cells within the tumor are in a stage of division.

Sarcoma — A form of cancer that arises in the supportive tissues such as bone, cartilage, fat or muscle.

Secondary Tumor — A tumor that develops as a result of metastasis or spreads beyond the original cancer.

Secondary Site — A second site in which cancer is found. Example: cancer in the lymph nodes near the breast is a secondary site.

Side Effects — Usually describes situations that occur after treatments. For example, hair loss may be a side effect of chemotherapy; fatigue may be a side effect of radiation therapy.

Staging — An evaluation of the extent of the disease, such as breast cancer. A classification based on stage at diagnosis which helps determine the appropriate treatment and prognosis. In breast cancer, the classification is determined by whether the lymph nodes are involved; whether the cancer has spread to other parts of the body (through the lymphatic system or bloodstream) and set up distant metastasis; and the size of the tumor. Five different stages (0-4) are used in breast cancer with levels in each stage. Stage IV is the most serious.

Stellate — Appearing on mammography as a star-shape because of the irregular growth of cells into surrounding tissue. May be associated with a malignancy or some benign conditions.

SHARING WITH OTHER BREAST CANCER PATIENTS IS VERY IMPORTANT. YOU CANNOT, MUST NOT, NEED NOT DO IT ALONE!

—*FELICIA SMITH*
Survivor

Stereotactic Needle Biopsy — A biopsy done while the breast is compressed under mammography. A series of pictures locate the lesion, and a radiologist enters information into a computer. The computer calculates information and positions a needle to remove the finding. A needle is inserted into the lump, and a piece of tissue is removed and sent to the lab for analysis. May be referred to as mammotest or core biopsy.

Stomatitis — Inflammation of the gastrointestinal tract creating discomfort and a potential for infection. May be caused by chemotherapy drugs.

Supraclavicular Nodes — The nodes located above the collarbone in the area of the neck.

T

Tamoxifen — An anti-estrogen drug that may be given to women with estrogen receptive tumors to block estrogen from entering the breast tissues. May produce menopause-like symptoms, including hot flashes and vaginal dryness. Currently being used with high risk women in clinical trials to prevent breast cancer and with women who have had breast cancer to prevent recurrence.

Thrombocytopenia — A decrease in the number of platelets in the blood, resulting in the potential for increased bleeding and decreased ability for clotting.

Tissue — A collection of similar cells. There are four basic types of tissues in the body: epithelial, connective, muscle and nerve.

Transillumination — The inspection of an organ by passing a light through the tissues. Transmission of the light varies with different densities.

Tumor — An abnormal tissue, swelling or mass, may be either benign or malignant.

Two-Step Procedure — When surgical biopsy and breast surgery are performed in two separate surgeries.

THE REALITY OF NO BREASTS MADE ME FEEL LIKE AN "IT." IT WAS TRULY SILENT SUFFERING. YET, NOW, I CAN TALK ABOUT IT, WHEN BEFORE, I WAS MORTIFIED.

—*Survivor*

U

Ultrasound Examination — The use of high frequency sound waves to locate a tumor inside the body. Helps determine if a breast lump is solid tissue or filled with fluids.

Ultrasound Guided Biopsy — The use of ultrasound to guide a biopsy needle to obtain a sample of tissue for analysis by a pathologist.

USE EVERY RESOURCE AVAILABLE TO YOU TO HELP YOU COPE WITH THE EMOTIONAL PAIN—FAMILY, FRIENDS, PEERS, SUPPORT GROUPS AND PROFESSIONAL COUNSELORS.

—Survivor

INDEX

Additional Resources
available from EduCareInc.com
1-800-849-9271

Helping Your Mate Face Breast Cancer . . .
Tips for Becoming an Effective Support Partner

Fully Revised 5th Edition

Helping Your Mate Face Breast Cancer is described as the essential "how-to" manual for support partners. It is a complete primer on disease and treatment options, sexual relationships after cancer, therapeutic communication guidelines and balancing daily living with the fear of recurrence. Illustrated procedures, a glossary and experiences from other partners make this book an invaluable resource for the support partner.

Finding a Lump in Your Breast —
Where To Go . . . What To Do

Fully Revised 2nd Edition

Finding A Lump In Your Breast — Where To Go . . . What To Do, instructs women on how to monitor their breast health. It is a practical guide designed to help women acquire a healthy knowledge of their breasts, understand common conditions that may occur and how to detect abnormal changes.

Solving the Mystery of Breast Pain

Fully Revised 2nd Edition

Solving the Mystery of Breast Pain offers women proactive steps to assess and manage breast pain. Instructional worksheets assist the woman and her physician to identify potential causes of pain. Included is a list of more than 400 prescription and over-the-counter medications, as well as common herbal products that may cause or promote breast pain.

Managing My Fears

List all the fears and worries you are presently facing. In the second column, list the name of the most appropriate person with whom to verbalize these fears. In the third column, think about and list things you can do to change or reduce these fears.

Fears	Person(s) Involved	Things I Can Do

"You can gain strength, courage, and confidence by every experience in which you really stop to look fear in the face.
The danger lies in refusing to face the fear, in not daring to come to grips with it. You must do something you think you cannot do."

— Eleanor Roosevelt

Managing My Fears

"To fight fear ACT.
To increase fear—
wait, put off, post-
pone."

— David Joseph
Schwartz

Fears	Person(s) Involved	Things I Can Do

Check the questions you would like to have answered.
Tear out this sheet and take it to your surgical consultation.

Surgeon's Name: _____   **Date:** _____

General Questions

- ☐ What is the name of the type of breast cancer I have?
- ☐ How large is the tumor?
- ☐ Is the tumor in situ (inside ducts or lobules) or invasive (grown through walls of ducts or lobules)?
- ☐ Do you expect cancer cells to be found in my lymph nodes?
- ☐ Do you expect that the cancer has invaded anything else (skin, muscle, bones, other organs)?
- ☐ Is there any evidence from my mammogram that there might be cancer anywhere else in this breast or in the opposite breast?
- ☐ Does my type of cancer have an increased risk of being found in the same breast or occurring, at a further time, in the opposite breast?

Additional Questions _____

_____

_____

Lumpectomy Questions

- ☐ Am I a candidate for a lumpectomy?
- ☐ If so, how do you expect my breast to appear after surgery, considering the size of the lump and tissue you need to remove compared to the size of my breast, or the position of the lump in the breast?
- ☐ Do you think the cosmetic results will be acceptable?
- ☐ Which of the lumpectomy procedures do you plan to use (segmental, tylectomy, lumpectomy)?
- ☐ Am I a candidate for sentinel lymph node biopsy?
  If so, do you evaluate the removed sentinel lymph node(s) during surgery or after surgery?
- ☐ Will you remove lymph nodes by a separate incision under my arm?
- ☐ What do you consider the advantages and disadvantages of a lumpectomy for my case?
- ☐ Will a lumpectomy give me the same chance for control of my cancer as a mastectomy?
- ☐ Will I need to have radiation therapy after a lumpectomy?
- ☐ How long will I be in the hospital?
- ☐ Will I have drains in the incision after surgery?
- ☐ Will I go home with drains?
- ☐ When do you expect the drains to be removed?
- ☐ How long will I need to be away from my job?

Additional Questions _____

_____

_____

Mastectomy Questions

☐ Which type of mastectomy do you plan to perform? (Refer to pages 31-33)

☐ What do you think are the advantages and disadvantages of having a mastectomy?

☐ In my particular case, does mastectomy offer a better chance of control of my cancer?

☐ Am I a candidate for sentinel lymph node biopsy?

   If so, do you evaluate the removed sentinel lymph node(s) during surgery or after surgery?

☐ How many and what levels of lymph nodes do you plan to remove?

☐ Will I have drain bulbs in my incision after surgery? If so, how many?

☐ Will I go home with drains in place?

☐ When are drains usually removed?

☐ Will I have to have stitches/sutures removed? When and where will this be done?

☐ How long will I be in the hospital?

☐ When should I be able to resume my normal activities?

☐ Are there any types of limitations that I should expect in my surgical arm in the future?

Additional Questions _____

_____

Reconstruction Questions

☐ Am I a candidate for immediate reconstruction?

☐ Can you provide me with information about immediate reconstruction?

☐ Tell me the advantages of immediate reconstruction. Tell me the disadvantages of immediate reconstruction.

☐ Could you provide me with information on the use of implants and the potential use of my body tissues for reconstruction?

☐ Do you foresee anything in my present health status which could prevent me from having either type of reconstruction?

Additional Questions _____

_____

Final Questions

☐ Is there anything else you need to tell me about my cancer or surgery?

☐ Do you have any written information on my cancer or surgery?

☐ Do you recommend any books or videos?

☐ Do you recommend any support groups or a professional counselor?

☐ If I have additional questions, whom should I call and whom should I speak with (nurse/physician)?

Additional Questions _____

_____

202

Tumor Location & Size

Tumor Location

Ask your physician to draw where your tumor is located in your breast and the estimated amount of tissue that will be removed during surgery.

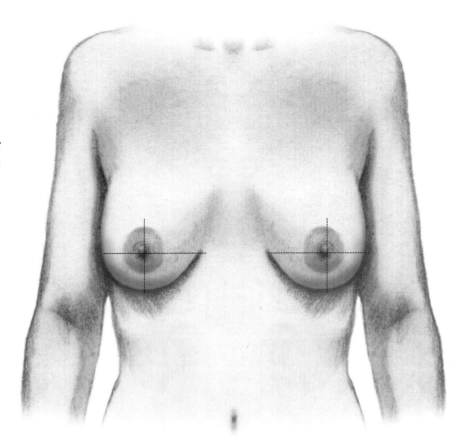

Tumor Size

Ask your physician to draw the estimated size of your tumor on this chart.

Tumor size is the largest dimension of the tumor. Results are reported in centimeters (cm) or millimeters (mm).

    10 mm equals 1 cm

    1 cm equals 3/8 inch

    1 inch equals 2.5 cm

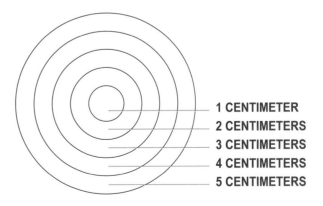

1 CENTIMETER
2 CENTIMETERS
3 CENTIMETERS
4 CENTIMETERS
5 CENTIMETERS

Appearance After Surgery

Ask your surgeon to draw your planned incision.

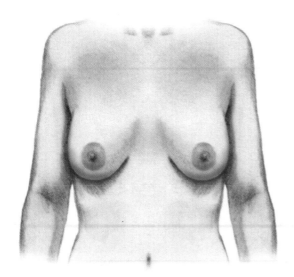

Lumpectomy Scar

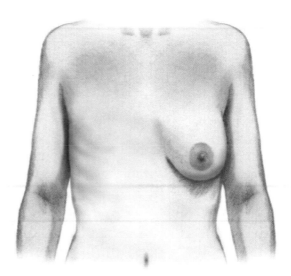

Right Mastectomy Scar

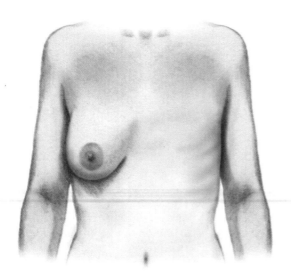

Left Mastectomy Scar

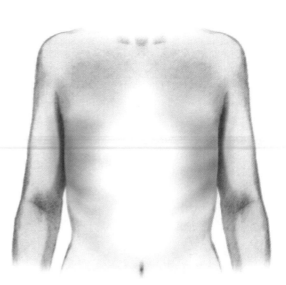

Bilateral Mastectomy Scars

Surgical Decision Evaluation

Answer the following questions to help uncover your true feelings. The statements are in pairs. Read both statements before you answer. **Choose only one answer between the two statements that best states how you feel at this time**. You will circle either an A or a B in the column on the right for each section.

A	I would **resent** losing my breast.	A B
B.	I would **accept** losing my breast.	
A.	My breasts are **very important** as to how I feel about my self-image.	A B
B.	My breasts are **not** that important as to how I feel about my self-image.	
A.	My goal is to **preserve** my body image (breast), if possible.	A B
B.	My goal is to **reduce** my **chances** of **local** recurrence (in breast) to the lowest level possible.	
A.	I **don't want** to lose my breast and be required to wear a prosthesis or have reconstructive surgery.	A B
B.	I would **rather** lose my breast to reduce the chance of recurrence to the lowest level.	
A.	I would, **without increased anxiety**, perform breast self-exam or go for clinical exams on the lumpectomy breast.	A B
B.	I would **worry** about recurrence in the remaining breast tissues after lumpectomy.	
A.	I'm **not a worrier**; I would see my doctor as needed.	A B
B.	**I would worry** about the cancer coming back in my remaining breast tissues.	
A.	I would **agree** to go to radiation therapy five days a week for five to seven weeks to save my breast.	A B
B.	I would rather **not** have to travel back to the hospital for five to seven weeks for radiation therapy.	
A.	I **don't mind** going to **radiation** for five to seven weeks to keep my breast.	A B
B.	I don't have time to keep going back to the hospital. **I want to get this over.**	
A.	To keep my breast, I could **accept changes** after radiation therapy such as increased lumpiness and a decrease in size.	A B
B.	I would **be anxious** about monitoring a breast that had lumpy changes after radiation.	
A.	These changes (lumpiness, change in size) are **minor** compared to not having my breast.	A B
B.	It would **overwhelm** me to feel my breast after having had cancer in it.	
A.	I feel that my breast is **important** to my sexuality and self esteem; without a breast I would feel less sexually attractive to my partner.	A B
B.	My partner does **not care** if I have a breast or not; our relationship would not change if I lost my breast.	
A.	I **do not think** I would ever feel sexy again without my breast.	A B
B.	I **do think** I could feel sexy again without my breast.	

Add the number of A and B's you selected. Total A's _____ Total B's _____

The highest number shows your inclination to prefer this type of surgical procedure.

A= Lumpectomy   B= Mastectomy

This is a guide, not the answer, as to your inclination toward surgical options.

Reconstruction Decision Evaluation

If your total for mastectomy had the higher number, or if you simply prefer mastectomy, you now need to consider your options for reconstructive surgery. Continue to choose between the two statements in the same manner.

A. I **would dislike** wearing an external prosthesis (breast form) daily. B. I **would rather** wear an external prosthesis than to have additional surgery.	A B
A. I **don't** want to have to wear a **prosthesis,** because it would be a daily reminder of having lost my breast to cancer. I want my body image to be back to normal as soon as possible. B. I would **do anything** to **avoid** additional surgery.	A B
A. I **do** want to be able to wear low-cut clothing or go braless. B. I **don't** want to wear low-cut clothing or go braless.	A B
A. I **don't** want to have to wear a prosthesis to maintain my body image. B. I **would rather** wear a prothesis than have more surgery.	A B

Add the number of A and B's you selected. Total A's _____ Total B's _____

Your inclination to prefer reconstruction or no reconstruction procedure.   **A= Reconstruction   B= Prosthesis**

Delayed or Immediate Reconstruction

A. I would **rather have time to recover** from my mastectomy and treatments before I have reconstructive surgery. B. I would **rather have all of my surgeries** performed at the time of my breast cancer surgery than to have to return after chemotherapy or radiation therapy.	A B
A. **Additional surgery** is **too much** to undergo when my anxiety is so high about my cancer. B. **Let's do it all now** and get it over with; I don't like putting things off that I need to do.	A B
A. I want to **take my time** finding a reconstructive surgeon and studying the different types of reconstructive surgery before I make a decision. B. I **understand** my reconstructive **options** and feel comfortable with the recommended reconstructive surgeon.	A B
A. Reconstructive surgery is too important to **make a fast decision** when I am overwhelmed about my cancer. B. Why should I have to **wait** to have my body image restored?	A B

Add the number of A and B's you selected. Total A's _____ Total B's _____

A = Delayed   B = Immediate Reconstruction

Remember, your decisions need to be made according to how **you feel** about the changes your surgical choice would have on you. Each option has advantages and disadvantages to consider. **Survival rates are equal.** Talk to a variety of healthcare professionals (surgeon, medical oncologist, radiation oncologist, plastic surgeon, nurse) and women about the types of surgeries to arrive at your final conclusion.

Questions For Reconstructive Surgeon

Check the questions you would like to have answered.
Tear out this sheet and take it to your reconstructive consultation.

Surgeon's Name _____ **Date** _____

☐ What type of surgery do you recommend for me?

☐ If autologous (my own body tissues) which type of surgery do you recommend? (See reverse side of this sheet for descriptions of surgery types.)

☐ Do you suggest use of my own body tissues or an implant?

☐ If an implant, what kind of implant do you recommend? Will it be placed under the muscle?

☐ What are the advantages and disadvantages of the recommended surgery?

☐ May I see photographs and talk to some of your patients?

☐ What can I expect to look like after surgery?

☐ Will you reconstruct my nipple and areola?

☐ How much feeling (sensation) will I have in my reconstructed breast?

☐ How will my breast feel when touched (soft, firm)?

☐ Will this surgery cause me to have additional scars?

☐ Will my surgery cause any restrictions on future physical activities (employment, sports or ability to exercise)?

☐ How many surgical procedures will my reconstruction require?

☐ How long will I be in surgery for each of these procedures?

☐ How long will I be in the hospital for each procedure?

☐ How often will I need a return appointment with you?

☐ How long will it take to complete the reconstruction process?

☐ How long before I can return to work or normal activities after each procedure?

☐ How much will it cost and how much should my insurance cover?

☐ In the future, what problems could potentially occur after reconstructive surgery?

Additional Questions _____

_____

_____

_____

_____

Reconstructive Surgery Options

TYPE	ADVANTAGES	DISADVANTAGES	INDICATIONS	CONTRAINDICATIONS
Tissue Expander and Implant	▪ Short surgical time ▪ Low cost	▪ Multiple fillings of expander with saline ▪ 2nd surgery for implant ▪ Capsular contracture ▪ Leakage or rupture	▪ Medium size breast (400 - 800 cc) ▪ Lumpectomy defect ▪ Tight skin from radiation therapy	▪ None ▪ Previous radiation therapy may limit size
Implant: Saline or Silicone	▪ Short surgical time ▪ One-step procedure ▪ Lower cost	▪ Capsular contracture ▪ Leakage or rupture ▪ Autoimmune disease (>.5%)	▪ Small breast (400 - 600 cc)	▪ Thin skin flaps ▪ Radiation therapy
Latissimus Dorsi Flap (Pedicle Flap) **Muscle and Tissue**	▪ Autologous tissue and muscle remain attached to blood supply ▪ Small donor scar	▪ Minor muscle weakness ▪ Potential seroma ▪ Flap necrosis	▪ Small to medium size breast (400 - 800 cc) ▪ Lumpectomy defect ▪ Tight skin from radiation therapy	▪ None
TAP Thoracodorsal Artery Perforator (Free Flap) Tissues Only	▪ Autologous tissue with blood vessels ▪ No muscle removed ▪ Small donor scar	▪ Potential seroma ▪ Flap necrosis	▪ Small to medium sized breast (400 - 800 cc) ▪ Lumpectomy defect ▪ Tight skin from radiation therapy	▪ Extremely thin women
TRAM Flap Transverse Rectus Abdominis Myocutaneous (Pedicle)	▪ Autologous muscle with tissues attached to local blood supply ▪ Tummy tuck	▪ Scar on abdomen ▪ Minor muscle weakness ▪ Extended operative time ▪ 6 - 12 wks. recovery ▪ Abdominal wall hernia ▪ Flap necrosis	▪ Mastectomy	▪ Previous abdominal surgery ▪ Physical condition ▪ Cigarette smokers (some physicians)
DIEP Deep Interior Epigastric Perforator (Free Flap)	▪ Abdominal tissues with blood vessels and nerves ▪ Potential return of nerve sensations in area	▪ Additional scar on abdomen ▪ Extended operative time from microscopic reattachment ▪ Flap necrosis	▪ Mastectomy	▪ Previous abdominal surgery ▪ Physical condition ▪ Cigarette smokers (some physicians) ▪ Extremely thin women
Inferior Gluteus Flap (Free Flap)	▪ Autologous tissues, muscle and blood vessels cut from lower buttocks	▪ Scar at donor site ▪ 6 - 12 weeks recovery ▪ Extended surgical reattachment time ▪ Flap necrosis	▪ Mastectomy	▪ Cigarette smokers (some physicians) ▪ Extremely thin women
S-GAP Superior Gluteal Artery Perforator (Free Flap)	▪ Autologous tissues, blood vessels, and nerves cut from upper buttocks ▪ Potential return of nerve sensation	▪ Scar at donor site ▪ Shorter recovery ▪ Extended surgical reattachment time ▪ Flap necrosis	▪ Mastectomy	▪ Cigarette smokers (some physicians) ▪ Extremely thin women

Personal Healthcare Provider Records

Primary Physician

Name

Telephone

Address

Nurse

Radiation Oncologist

Name

Telephone

Address

Nurse

Surgeon

Name

Telephone

Address

Nurse

Plastic Surgeon

Name

Telephone

Address

Nurse

Oncologist

Name

Telephone

Address

Nurse

Breast Health Educator

Name

Telephone

Address

Personal Healthcare Provider Records

Breast Health Center

Name

Telephone

Address

Hospital

Name

Telephone

Address

Pharmacy

Name

Telephone

Address

Social Worker

Name

Telephone

Address

Support Group

Name

Telephone

Address

Other

Name

Telephone

Address

Personal Treatment Record

Name _____

Baseline Vital Signs _____

Blood Pressure _____ Pulse _____ Respirations _____ Weight _____

Allergies _____

Routine Medications _____

Date of Diagnosis _____ Date of Surgery _____

Diagnosis _____ Size of Tumor _____ Node Status _____

ER/PR Status _____ Other Tests _____

Baseline Vital Signs _____

Name of Chemotherapy Drugs	Chemotherapy Treatment	Radiation Therapy	Hormonal Treatment
_____	Start Date _____	Start Date _____	Start Date _____
_____	_____	_____	_____
_____	_____	_____	_____
_____	_____	_____	_____
_____	_____	_____	_____
_____	_____	_____	_____
_____	_____	_____	_____
_____	_____	_____	_____
_____	_____	_____	_____
_____	_____	_____	_____
_____	Completion	Completion	Completion

Chemotherapy Treatment Notes

_____

_____

_____

_____

_____

_____

_____

_____

_____

_____

Dates of Treatment

_____

_____

_____

_____

_____

_____

_____

_____

_____

_____

_____

Drain Bulb Record

Measure and record drainage of bulb(s) each time you empty drain.
Take this record to your physician.

Date	Time	Drain 1	Drain 2	Total

Drain Bulb Record

Measure and record drainage of bulb(s) each time you empty drain.
Take this record to your physician.

Date	Time	Drain 1	Drain 2	Total

Hospital Discharge Instructions

Prior to leaving the hospital, your nurse will provide you with verbal and written instructions concerning your care and a list of symptoms that might occur and need to be reported to the doctor. During your hospitalization, it may be helpful to write down any questions as they occur. When your doctor makes the final hospital visit, you may want to be prepared to clarify the following. Check the questions you wish to have answered.

- ☐ If you do not remember what your doctor said about your surgery or diagnosis the day you had surgery, ask for clarification.

- ☐ What activities should I avoid until my next appointment?

- ☐ Are there any special exercises or recommendations regarding the use of my arm?

- ☐ Will the numbness, tingling or sensations experienced be temporary or permanent?

- ☐ What type of pain is normal after my type of surgery?

- ☐ What medications will I take for pain?

- ☐ Will I be given any prescriptions for medication to take home?

- ☐ Do I resume previous medications (especially estrogen-type medications)?

- ☐ When can I shampoo my hair?

- ☐ When can I shower or take a tub bath?

- ☐ When can I remove my bandage?

- ☐ When can I drive?

- ☐ When do I need make my next appointment?

- ☐ Will I be referred to any other doctors or have any other treatments?

- ☐ If so, when will I see these doctors? Who will make the appointments?

- ☐ When will my pathology report be available?

- ☐ Is there anything that I can do to ensure a speedy recovery?

Ask your nurse to write down any appointment dates or names of doctors that you will be referred to for further evaluation concerning treatment.

Additional Questions _____

_____

_____

_____

_____

_____

Questions For Medical Oncologist Worksheet

Check the questions you would like to have answered.
Tear out this sheet and take it to your appointment with the oncologist.

Oncologist's Name: _____ **Date:** _____

My Treatment:
- ☐ What kind of treatment will I receive (chemotherapy, hormonal, immunotherapy)?
- ☐ On what schedule will I receive these treatments?
- ☐ How long will I receive treatments?
- ☐ How long will each treatment take?
- ☐ Where will I receive my treatments (office, clinic, hospital)?
- ☐ Will any other tests be given before or while I receive my chemotherapy?
- ☐ Can someone come with me when I receive my treatments?
- ☐ Will I feel like driving myself home after my treatment or do I need a driver?
- ☐ Will I need radiation therapy?
- ☐ Do you have written information on my cancer or treatment plans?

Preparing for My Treatments:
- ☐ Should I eat before I come for my treatments?
- ☐ Can I take vitamins or herbs if I so choose?
- ☐ What kind of protection precautions to my skin should I take during chemotherapy (exposure to sunlight)?

After My Treatments:
- ☐ What side effects will I experience from the treatments (nausea, hair loss, changes in blood cell counts, etc.)?
- ☐ Will I be given medications to treat the side effects?
- ☐ When I complete my treatments, how often will I return for checkups?
- ☐ How will you evaluate the effectiveness of the treatments?

My Medications:
- ☐ What are the names of the drugs?
- ☐ Are the drugs given by mouth or into a vein?
- ☐ Will I need a port (device implanted under the skin) to receive any I.V. medications or will you use a vein in my arm?

Changes in My Body and Life:
- ☐ Will I continue to have menstrual periods? If not, when will they return?
- ☐ Should I use birth control? What type do you recommend?
- ☐ Will I be able to conceive and bear a child after treatment?
- ☐ What physical changes should I report to you or to your nurse during treatment?
- ☐ Can I continue my usual work or exercise schedules, or will I need to modify them during treatments?
- ☐ Are there any precautions my family should take to limit exposure to the chemotherapy during my treatments (shared eating utensils, bathroom facilities)?

Additional Questions _____

_____   _____

Medical Oncology Consultation Notes

Questions For Radiation Oncologist

Check the questions you would like to have answered.
Tear out this sheet and take it to your radiation consultation.

Physician's Name: _____ **Date:** _____

☐ How many radiation treatments will I receive?

☐ How long will my first visit take to mark the area?

☐ How do you mark the area that will be radiated?

☐ What kind of soap and bath do you recommend during my treatments?

☐ Is there anything that I cannot use during my treatment (deodorant, perfume, lotions to the chest or back, etc.)?

☐ Can I wear a bra or my prosthesis during radiation treatments?

☐ Do you have written information on radiation therapy for the breast area?

☐ What side effects are considered normal during radiation therapy?

☐ What side effects, if they occur, should I report immediately?

☐ In the future, what changes could potentially occur in the radiated breast?

Additional Questions _____

_____

_____

_____

_____

_____

_____

_____

_____

_____

Radiation Oncology Consultation Notes

Patient Appointment Reminder   Worksheet

Next Scheduled Appointment

Physician _____ **Date** _____ **Time** _____

It is helpful to write down questions for your nurse or physician prior to your visit.
It is also helpful to keep a list of thoughts which need to be communicated to your healthcare team.

Questions to ask physician _____

_____

_____

_____

_____

_____

_____

_____

Questions to ask nurse _____

_____

_____

_____

_____

_____

_____

_____

Remember to tell physician/nurse _____

_____

_____

_____

_____

_____

_____

Patient Appointment Reminder

Next Scheduled Appointment

Physician _____ **Date** _____ **Time** _____

It is helpful to write down questions for your nurse or physician prior to your visit.
It is also helpful to keep a list of thoughts which need to be communicated to your healthcare team.

Questions to ask physician _____

_____
_____
_____
_____
_____
_____
_____

Questions to ask nurse _____

_____
_____
_____
_____
_____
_____

Remember to tell physician/nurse _____

_____
_____
_____
_____
_____
_____
_____

Exercise Guidelines After Breast Cancer   Worksheet

Physician _____   **Date** _____

It is proven that a regular program of walking during breast cancer treatment can significantly increase the quality of life for a patient. However, it is important to get your physician's approval before starting this or any exercise program.

Recommended Walking Exercise Program:

Frequency: 4 times a week minimum, 6 times a week maximum; try not to skip more than 1 day in a row if your health allows

Goal: Gradually increase and maintain your heart rate at 100 to 120 beats/minute during walking

Place: Outdoors preferably when weather permits; indoor mall or treadmill

Attire: Comfortable shoes designed for walking; layered, loose, cotton clothing to absorb perspiration; and carry personal identification in case of an emergency

Recommended Routine:

1. 5 minutes slow walking to warm up.

2. Increase walking to brisk pace to increase heart rate to 100 to 120 beats per minute (take your pulse for 6 seconds and multiply by 10 to check your heart rate).

3. Gradually increase the time your pulse remains at your target heart rate by extending your walk as tolerated. Walking should increase your energy after your heart rate returns to normal, without causing fatigue. Do not exercise to a point of causing fatigue; this is not healthy nor recommended.

4. Last 5 minutes, reduce pace to allow your heart rate to gradually return to normal.

Do not exercise if you have:

- Fever
- Nausea or vomiting
- Muscle pain, joint pain or swelling
- Bleeding from any source
- Irregular heart beat
- Dizziness or fainting
- Chest, arm or jaw pain
- Intravenous chemotherapy administration on same day
- Blood drawing on same day—may exercise afterward; prior exercise may alter counts
- Any restrictions placed on exercise activities by a physician

Exercise Precautions During Treatment:

If you are receiving chemotherapy, your nurse/physician will alert you if your counts are in a range where exercise is not advised. When you have your blood drawn ask the nurse if your counts are still in a safe range.

Recommendations not to exercise are as follows:

1. White blood count less than 3,000 mm^3

2. Absolute granulocyte count less than 2,500 mm^3

3. Hemoglobin/hematocrit less than 10g/dl

4. Platelet count less than 25,000 mm^3

Exercise Tips:

- Walk with a partner, if possible

- Carry identification with you

- Listen to inspirational tapes or your favorite music, if you walk alone

- Keep an exercise log or diary to monitor your progress

- Walk at the same time each day if possible to make walking a routine

- Drink a full glass of water before and after your walk

- Walk in a safe area, away from traffic

Exercise During Treatment:

Exercise during treatments—chemotherapy or radiation therapy—has to be self-paced. Only you can determine how much you can tolerate and when you feel up to exercising. Begin at a modest level and gradually increase your length of time. Take into consideration that during treatment there may be periods of decreased performance due to effects of treatment. Do not push yourself during these times. A walking exercise program can be easily modified to meet your changing needs during treatment; it can be started, suspended, decreased, or accelerated according to your physical energy. You may also want to consider other types of exercise such as biking, swimming or gardening.

Check with your physician to determine if this walking program or any other exercise program is recommended during your recovery. Clinical studies have proven that women who walked four to five times weekly during treatments, for 20 to 45 minutes, had more energy; experienced less depression, nausea, and insomnia; gained less weight; and required less medication to control side effects of treatment than women who did not exercise. An exercise program is one thing you can do to promote your own recovery while you are still in treatment.

My Commitment to an Exercise Program:

I will check with my doctor about starting my walking program: (date) _____

I am starting an exercise program: (date) _____

I am going to ask (person) to join me: _____

I am going to keep a record of my walking program: (yes/no)_____

I plan to walk: (place) _____

Items I need to start my walking exercise program: (shoes, shorts, shirts, tape or CD player, tapes or CDs, radio, I-Pod): ___

_____

_____

_____

Relaxation Response Guidelines

Learning The Relaxation Response —The Stress Controller For Better Health

The diagnosis of breast cancer is a very stressful event. After the diagnosis, a continual series of events cause fear and increases stress. The list of additional stressors that cancer brings goes on and on—surgical choices, chemotherapy, radiation therapy, side effects of treatment, changes in family and changes in work. A limited amount of stress is helpful and serves as motivation. But the constant stress after a breast cancer diagnosis can become a major contributor to physical and mental fatigue. This fatigue and stress can decrease the quality of your life and slow your recovery.

A fearful or stressed body has the "fight-or-flight" response. Our bodies prepare to fight or to run from our attackers. During this time of stress or fear, our heart rate increases, our breathing rate increases, our blood pressure increases, our metabolic rate increases and our muscles become tense. Researchers have concluded that chronic arousal of the fight-or-flight state may lead to permanent physiological changes—disease. They have also found that the stress reaction can be altered by practicing relaxation techniques.

The most well-known researcher of relaxation's effects on the body is Dr. Herbert Benson of Harvard Medical School. Dr. Benson's thirty years of research at Harvard has proven that a person can consciously reverse this fight-or-flight stress by learning the "relaxation response" when faced with fears and stressors. (Recommended for additional information: *Relaxation Response* by Dr. Herbert Benson, William Morrow Publishing, 1975; *The Wellness Book: A Comprehensive Guide to Maintaining Health and Treating Stress-Related Illness*, Dr. Herbert Benson, Fireside Publishing, 1993.)

The relaxation response decreases the respiratory rate, heart rate, blood pressure, metabolism rate and muscle tension in the body. In other words, the relaxation response is a built-in method of stress control. It can interrupt the fight-or-flight response and the negative effects it produces in your body when you become tense or fearful. It is a method of stress control that you can learn and practice anywhere, anytime. It will not cost you anything and has no negative side effects.

During treatment for breast cancer, you may face many things which cause you to become stressed and fearful, creating the fight-or-flight effects in your body. You need a plan to free yourself from the stress of your environment to develop a state of relaxation. The state of relaxation, allows your body to return to the state that is most conducive for recovery. Dr. Benson's techniques for learning to relax, even during stressful or fearful times, can give you the power to remain in control of your physiological response to an event.

How do you learn to relax? It begins with a conscious effort.

- Find a quiet room away from interruptions and sit up straight in a chair
- Place your hands comfortably in your lap
- Close your eyes
- Select a phrase, prayer or word that gives you a sense of peace, love and safety*
- Take a deep breath very slowly and hold it for a few seconds
- As you breathe out slowly, repeat the phrase or word
- Continue inhaling and exhaling while repeating your phrase for 10 to 20 minutes
- When your mind wanders to another thought, refuse to entertain it and gently bring your thoughts back to your breathing and repetitive phrase
- Open your eyes and gradually re-orient yourself to your surroundings

During relaxation you may feel changes in sensations such as a tingling, a sense of floating, drifting or dropping. This indicates that your body is relaxing; it is returning to a state that allows physical recovery to be optimized. It is suggested that the relaxation response be practiced twice a day or used at anytime you feel stressed or fearful.

Mini Relaxation Responses

Often there are times when stressful situations arise when we need to gain control but we cannot leave our environment for a quiet place. Simply decide to concentrate on breathing and repeating your phrase with your eyes open, if necessary. Taking a deep breath increases the oxygen to the brain and clears the thinking. Focusing on a word or phrase* during this time of concentrated breathing interrupts the anxiety that the situations produce. Doing a mini relaxation response can break the tendency to become over-stressed during an event such as having an IV puncture inserted, going through a diagnostic test, undergoing a new procedure or taking chemotherapy or radiation. Utilize your ability to manage stress, keeping your body in a more relaxed state, by practicing the mini relaxation response anytime, anywhere.

*Suggested Words or Phrases:

Select a word or phrase that gives you a sense of peace from this list or choose one of your own not listed.

General: Love, Peace, Calm, Relax, Healing

Christian: "Our Father who art in heaven" — "The Lord is my shepherd" — "Lord, Jesus Christ, have mercy on me"

Jewish: "Sh'ma Yisroel" — "Shalom" — "The Lord is my shepherd"

Visualization Relaxation

Another technique is to replace the repetitive phrase with a mental picture of a scene that brings a sense of peace and safety—a garden, park, seashore, etc. As you breathe slowly, mentally feel and explore the beauty of this favorite place in your mind—smell the fragrances, feel the warmth of the sun, hear the familiar sounds. Visualization also promotes the relaxation response in your body.

Taking charge of stress and keeping it manageable is a step toward improving mental and physical health. Learning to relax is something you can do to remain in control of your emotions during times of stress, preventing the fight-or-flight response, and creating an environment for your optional recovery.

Personal Plan For Recovery

Take the time to plan steps of action in every area of your life for maximum recovery. Inventory your life and make the adjustments you feel will restore a sense of control.

Support System

Personal: Identify at least two people you can talk to openly.

I can talk to: _____ and _____

Information: Identify sources of correct information on breast cancer.
Check the resource section of this book.

Physician: _____ phone: _____

Physician: _____ phone: _____

Nurse: _____ phone: _____

Organization: _____ phone: _____

Organization: _____ phone: _____

Organization: _____ phone: _____

Organization: _____ phone: _____

Support: Identify your local support groups by calling the American Cancer Society.

Breast Cancer Patients: _____ phone: _____

Mate's Groups: _____ phone: _____

Children's Classes: _____ phone: _____

Spiritual: Identify people who can help you deal with the spiritual aspects of your illness.

_____ phone: _____

_____ phone: _____

_____ phone: _____

"Planning is like a road map.

It can show us the way and head us in the right direction and keep us on course.

Planning means mapping out how to get from here to where we want to be.

Planning is the power tool for achievement, the magic bridge to our goals and our success."

— Wynn Davis

227

☐ **Fears:** Name your fears and plan steps of action to address them. Complete the Fear Management worksheet on page 199.

☐ **Diet:** Evaluate your diet.

I plan to make the following changes: _____

☐ **Exercise:** Plan a program of exercise to restore and maintain your physical condition.

I plan to: _____

☐ **Personal Appearance:** Make plans to enhance your self-esteem and personal appearance during treatment.

I plan to: _____

☐ **Time Management:** Plan to make lifestyle changes: (Employment, Social, Civic duties)

I plan to start: _____

I plan to stop: _____

☐ **Family Management:** Make changes in your household.

I need to delegate chores for: _____

I need to hire help for: _____

I need to stop doing: _____

☐ **Personal Fulfillment:** Think of things you want to do more of or things you want to begin to do. Think selfishly. You deserve it!

I want to to add the following goals, hobbies or pleasurable events to my life.

I plan to: _____

_____

_____

☐ **Reaching Out:** A spirit of gratefulness and an effort on your part to help others is very rewarding.
Plan to say "thank you" to those who play an important part in your life and recovery.
Plan to give back to others who are in need.

People to write or thank: _____

Things I would like to do to help others: _____

Congratulations!
You have just taken steps to plan your psychological and social recovery.
Refer to this sheet when in doubt of what you can do to speed your recovery.

My Prayer During Breast Cancer

Lord, I have just received the diagnosis of breast cancer.

Still my anxious heart as I seek to understand why.

Teach me to transform my suffering into growth.

My great fear of tomorrow into faith in your presence.

My tears into understanding.

My discouragement into courage.

My anger into forgiveness.

My bitterness into acceptance.

My experience with cancer into my testimony.

My crisis into a platform on which

I can learn to help others.

God grant that one day I can embrace this time

as my friend, and not as my enemy.

— *Judy Kneece, RN, OCN*

What Cancer Can't Do

Cancer is so limited . . .

It cannot cripple love.

It cannot shatter hope.

It cannot corrode faith.

It cannot eat away peace.

It cannot destroy confidence.

It cannot kill friendship.

It cannot shut out memories.

It cannot silence courage.

It cannot invade the soul.

It cannot reduce eternal life.

It cannot quench the Spirit.

It cannot lessen the power of the resurrection.

— *Anonymous*

Cancer Can't Rob Me

Today is another new day and I can choose to use it in many ways. I did not choose to have cancer, but I can choose how I am going to respond and what I plan to do with today. Today is mine to make choices. This day can be a new beginning for me, if I so choose.

Today can be the day that I decide to exchange those things which weigh my spirit down for a lighter load of faith and trust. I can change my perception of cancer as a "robber" of my health and my future and exchange it into a vehicle to transport me into a life rich in understanding. This understanding will strengthen me and make me valuable to others who will walk the same path after me.

I can choose:

- To see cancer as a "challenge" instead of as a defeat.
- To demystify cancer by learning about my disease rather than cowering in fear of the unknown.
- To give up concentrating on the "things I can't control" and replace them with thoughts of "what I can control."
- To respond with a spirit of "I can" instead of "I can't."
- To ask for help and not try to face the challenge alone.
- To face my fears with a plan for steps of action against them.
- To look for the blessings in the events of today instead of focusing on losses.
- To add to my life the things I have always wanted to do but postponed until the right time.

Today is the time:

- To use my spiritual faith as a vehicle to understand why and give me hope.
- To let go of anger, bitterness and resentments, which only slow down my recovery.
- To see my cancer experience as a new tool for personal growth.
- To offer my support and share what I'm learning with others who may need my help.

Therefore, I choose for today:

Peace and not anxiety,

Good and not evil,

Love and not hate,

Gain and not loss.

When today becomes tomorrow, this day will

be gone forever leaving in its place what I choose today.

I, alone, can choose to use today wisely

— Cancer Can't Rob Me Of This Day!

Judy C. Kneece, RN, OCN

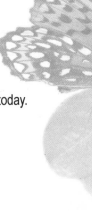